ANXiETY

Self Development Guide to Overcoming Anxiety,
Fear and Depression Through Cognitive
Behavioral Therapy

(Be Resilient and Recover From Ptsd)

Rick William

Published by Kevin Dennis

© **Rick William**

All Rights Reserved

Anxiety: Self Development Guide to Overcoming Anxiety,
Fear and Depression Through Cognitive Behavioral
Therapy (Be Resilient and Recover From Ptsd)

ISBN 978-1-989920-39-8

Legal & Disclaimer

The information contained in this book is not designed to replace or take the place of any form of medicine or professional medical advice. The information in this book has been provided for educational and entertainment purposes only.

The information contained in this book has been compiled from sources deemed reliable, and it is accurate to the best of the Author's knowledge; however, the Author cannot guarantee its accuracy and validity and cannot be held liable for any errors or omissions. Changes are periodically made to this book. You must consult your doctor or get professional medical advice before using any of the suggested remedies, techniques, or information in this book.

Upon using the information contained in this book, you agree to hold harmless the Author from and against any damages, costs, and expenses, including any legal fees potentially resulting from the application of any of the

Table of Contents

Introduction

Life is full of stress, and these days, it's so easy to fall into the traps of depression and anxiety. When that happens, you might feel like your life right now isn't good at all—and that you'd rather go back to the past because it's where your happiness lies.

That way of thinking is wrong. In fact, there are so many things you could do to help you forget about your worries, live in the present, and let go of anxiety and stress. You can start taking care of your mind—and mindfulness is a good start.

By reading this book, you will learn more about mindfulness, understand what mindfulness is about, why it's important, why eating and drinking slowly is important, how you can live a life free of stress and anxiety—and so much more!

Read this book now and find out how.

Thanks again for downloading this book, I hope you enjoy it!

Gratitude

Have you ever found yourself in a wonderful situation, but you still ended up thinking about what was missing or how the situation could be "better"? This is an incredibly common experience. We may have a great job, wealth, a lovely partner, and amazing children, but almost all of our attention is still given to thoughts about what we want to improve. We may be looking at a beautiful view, and instead of just enjoying it, we often end up thinking, "This would be perfect if... my soul mate was here, it was sunnier, or I had my camera." We may have a wonderful partner, and instead of recognizing that, we focus on how she can improve. Our minds are too busy thinking about what isn't "good enough" in our lives or what "could be better" to be grateful and appreciative of what we have. This typically the case even when we can admit our lives are wonderful.

But in any moment that we don't have or believe our thoughts that say, "Something isn't good enough," what remains is gratitude for what we have. Strangely enough, this is the experience we generally hope to achieve by trying to make life match our concept of "perfect."

Appreciation

Another common side effect of experiencing the present moment is that we naturally appreciate and enjoy the simple things. We can be completely captured by the smell of a flower, the beauty of a tree, the sound of a child's laugh, the elegance of a landscape, the wonder of modern technology, the taste of a potato chip, or anything else. When our attention isn't on thoughts, this appreciation arises naturally.

Most of us can walk on a path every day and never notice the trees, the design of the houses, the texture of the path, the smell of the plants, or the sounds of the birds. The reason we rarely take notice of these sounds, sights, and smells in our daily lives is that our attention is almost continuously on our own thoughts of past and future. Even if we do look at a tree, our attention is on our judgments, labels, and commentary about the tree rather than on the tree itself. Our attention is on our thoughts about what we witness rather than just experiencing what we witness purely through our senses. When our attention is taken off thoughts, we naturally notice and appreciate so many simple things in our daily life that we never experienced before.

The ability to experience the awe of something simple arises at the moments when we have silence or space between our thoughts. It is like seeing something for the first time. This feeling is similar to the sense of wonder and innocent curiosity that young children have.

Peace, relaxation, and completion

Any feeling of insufficiency, unworthiness, or unlovability is created by thoughts. Therefore, we naturally don't experience these feelings when we don't have, or don't believe, the thoughts that create them. When we are present, we feel loved, approved of, completely worthy, and lovable, and we feel that nothing is missing from our lives. We feel complete not because we have thoughts that say, "Everyone loves me," or "I am great," but because we don't have, or don't believe, the thoughts that make us feel unlovable, unworthy, or incomplete.

Without our thoughts to create our unhappiness, we feel content right now. Since we are already happy, we no longer feel a constant need or pull to improve ourselves, others, and our situation just to try to make ourselves happy. This feeling is like "aaaaahh, I can rest now." We feel that our life is complete. We can still pursue any of our goals, but our pursuit will no longer contain the idea that we need to achieve our goal in order to make ourselves happy. This eliminates our anxiety because there is no downside to not achieving the goal—we are already happy.

We may not realize it, but thinking takes up a lot of our energy, tightens our muscles, and weighs us down. For example, you can see for yourself right now how thinking tightens your muscles by checking to see if your tongue is pressed against the roof of your mouth or if your teeth are clenched together. If so, let your tongue and teeth drop, and feel how your face softens. When we are present, our whole body softens and relaxes; it feels as if a huge weight that we never knew we had has been lifted off our shoulders, and we are left with an abundance of energy.

Normally, our decisions on what to say and do are based on thoughts. We decide what to do based on our ideas of what we "should" do, our beliefs about what will make us happy, and our beliefs about what will make us suffer (our fears). When we choose what we "should" do, we are choosing what society has decided is the "right" way instead of doing what feels true and natural to us. When we use our thoughts to make decisions, we often decide to stay in situations that we don't enjoy because our thoughts make us fear change. Since our thoughts are all inherently based on the past, if we listen to our thoughts on how to act, we are basing our decisions on the past instead of allowing ourselves to follow what feels true at this moment.

Can you think of a time when you realized that your boyfriend or girlfriend was not right for you at all, and at that moment, you realized that you had known this all along? Many times, at the moment that we acknowledge that a job, a lover, or a situation isn't right for us, we also notice that we had always known that something wasn't right about it. What happens at this moment is that we remember or become aware that our intuition had been trying to tell us what to do, but we just hadn't been listening.

When we pay more attention to our intuition and learn to trust it, we can make the decision that feels right to us from the start rather than waiting months or years to recognize what we had truly always known.

With each passing year, you learned more and more concepts of what is "good" and "bad," thereby adding and believing more and more psychological thoughts. With each new concept you learned, it was as if someone were throwing one more of these plastic circles onto your glasses. As you believed more concepts of "good" and "bad," the amount of time that your mind was silent between thoughts got smaller and smaller. Eventually, you get to the point where your mind becomes crowded with so many thoughts that you very rarely get a break from them. As one circle slides away from the hole on the glasses, another takes its place almost instantly. Your attention goes from one thought to another with almost no silence in between. Therefore, you have very little experience of the present moment.

Since we are used to the action of believing thoughts, and we constantly do it automatically, it may seem as though the present moment is a temporary experience created by the action of disbelieving thoughts. However, if we don't commit the act of believing a thought (don't color in the circle), we are already present. When we disbelieve a thought, it is as if we are simply erasing the color of a circle that we just colored in, allowing us to see life as it is. We are essentially reversing our previous action. We wouldn't say that erasing the color of the circle is creating the uncolored transparency of the circle or the clearness of the spot on our lens. The circle has always been transparent, and the spot has always been empty—it's just that we've rarely gotten to experience this because we automatically and unconsciously go from believing one thought to another with almost no break. The experience of the present moment is quite simply what remains when no thought arises in our mind, or we don't engage in the action of believing a thought.

The experience of the present moment is what we have been searching for. Now, we will take a look at why our pursuit of happiness has not been effective at providing us with the peace and happiness that we want ...

Chapter 1: What Is Anxiety?

"The rest of your life will not be mastered in just one day

Relax and master the day

Then keep doing that every single day."

What to know about Anxiety?

Anxiety is caused by any stress you are going through. It is a feeling of dread which overcomes you about a future event. Nearly 30% of adults experience anxiety at some point in their lives. Anxiety disorders are treatable. With the right treatment, it could lead to a productive and healthy lifestyle by overcoming your anxiety.

Anxiety has a number of symptoms which are: irrational worry, distress, and fear. Anxiety can also overcome a person gradually. It usually occurs in anticipation of a stressful situation. Anxiety disorder is when you experience these feelings on an extreme level and they interfere with your daily life. This jittery feeling on a small scale is normal for everybody, but if they last typically more than six months or so, then they could be due to a disorder.

You experience irrational fear all the time and what motivated you to do something better or be prepared more has turned into a huge distraction. Anxiety, if left untreated could take a turn for the worse. It starts off with you being unmotivated and then outright stop doing things you once enjoyed. Then it leads to an inability to do normal tasks without a feeling of fear.

Anxiety can affect a person at any age. It is more common in women than men, according to the American psychiatric association.

Anxiety is a natural response of the body since the early days where man was all about survival. The onset of triggers for dangers allowed us to undertake necessary action on whether to fight or hide. Anxiety sets off many alarms in our body where we can physically feel the tension of the prevailing situation. Sweating and racing-heartbeat are common symptoms that allow being better in tune with the surrounding. This feeling of danger releases adrenaline which is a chemical of the brain that triggers acute stress response of our body. This response is also called the fight or flight response. It is a psychological reaction that occurs due to a perceived threat to survival or dangerous situation.

For us humans now, things have developed manifold. We are not running for our lives. We don't need a trigger of our fight or flight response while going about our daily activities. The nervous or anxious feeling before something important is a testament to our ancient survival tactic.

Anxiety has several levels. It could be mild, moderate, or severe, mostly ranging from jittery feeling to extreme fear. Panic attacks are always on a serious level where you are not able to focus on anything else. Your body will basically be on fight or flight mode. It is one of the most common forms of emotional disorder.

How you experience anxiety could be totally different from the other person. Some people have nightmares while others have to sit through a barrage of painful memories or thoughts. All in all, it is very exhausting in whatever shape or form anxiety affects a person. Some of the general symptoms are:

•Rapid breaths

•Nausea

•A headache or trouble in focusing

•Insomnia

•Increase in heart rate

This funny feeling called anxiety could be a lifesaver if it comes and goes at the right time. If it decides to stay, then it could be very harmful to the mental health of a person.

Unfortunately, the causes of anxiety are unknown as of yet. A lot of factors directly contribute to it though. Development of a person from their childhood is a huge factor. There could be a mishandled event which led to the development of anxiety. Psychological, environmental, and genetics are also some factors. Anxiety disorders can run in the family also.

What to know about Panic Attacks?

A panic attack is an unexpected and intense feeling of overwhelming fear. They entail various physical symptoms as well such as racing heartbeat, nausea, and the shortage of breath. A panic attack is a frightening experience both mentally and physically. Physically, panic attacks can cause your knees to go weak and have chest pain. It can also cause dizziness, and for a second you may think you are having a heart attack. It only lasts for a while, but it can leave you really terrified and wary that another one might be coming in the future.

When this situation keeps on happening frequently, then it is classified as a panic disorder. A panic disorder can cause a person to avoid a certain situation for the fear of panic attacks. They will eventually realize it is not the situation they were avoiding but the panic attack itself.

Lately, panic attacks have been categorized into expected and unexpected types by (DSM-5) Diagnostic and Statistical Manual of Mental Disorders. ("DSM-5 Criteria for Diagnosing Panic Disorder", 2019)[1].

•Expected panic attacks are usually caused by external stress factors, such as phobias.

•Unexpected ones don't have an obvious identifiable cause.

Panic and anxiety attack may seem similar because they share a lot of emotional and physical symptoms. It is difficult to differentiate between them sometimes.

You can also experience both at the same time. An example of it is, if you are experiencing anxiety about a stressful event, it will wind up into panic attacks on the arrival of the said event. Main differences are that panic attacks are mostly out of the blue. Anxiety could be due to an upcoming situation that you deem stressful or threatening.

A panic attack is different from an anxiety attack. Here are some symptoms of an anxiety attack:

•Dizziness

•Dry mouth

•Sweating

•Chills or hot flashes

•Worry and fear

•Restlessness

•Numbness

If you learn to manage your anxiety, then you can further go on to completely avoid a panic attack. There are many techniques to calm your mind and body whenever you notice that a panic attack may be arising. The oncoming symptoms will eventually fade away and you would have successfully avoided a panic attack.

Coping with a panic attack

Coping with the feeling of panic is the first step to manage panic attack successfully.

Some anxiety managing techniques are here below; they will not only help in warding off the panic attack but also successfully take control of the anxious feeling.

Focus on Breathing

The first step to take is to focus on and regulate your breathing. Irregular breathing can make your symptoms even worse. Take a count of slow and deep breaths to help calm yourself.

Stop your train of thoughts

Whatever is going on your mind, try and put a halt on them. Throw them out of the metaphorical window. Only focus on yourself and put yourself in control of your own thoughts.

Positive thoughts

Assign your mind a happy place to wander into whenever you are in the situation. It will help you eventually realize that nothing is as bad as it seems right now.

Put yourself first

Don't feel bad about asking for help or leaving the situation. If you deem it necessary at that time to help you, then don't second guess yourself.

Practice these strategies if you have symptoms of anxiety. You won't get efficient with dealing right away as it is a gradual process.

Confronting your fear is very important. Don't let fear of a panic attack control you. Ride out the attack because, in the end, you will know that nothing life threatening happened. It can help you understand the situation better.

Having someone close will also help; someone that can steadily assure you throughout it. These situations once experienced will help mentally prepare you better for these episodes until you finally learn to overcome it.

Stress, Depression, and Anxiety

Anxiety and depression are related to each other. If you have the former disorder, you will be likely to have depression as well. They can occur separately too.

If a person ignores anxiety and depression throughout their life, it will likely result in a physical health issue. Mostly heart-related problems arise due to untreated anxiety or depression.

What happens to the brain during anxiety?

Let's take the help of science to understand anxiety better. Brain chemistry also plays a vital role. Researchers believe that as a result of anxiety, the area of the brain in charge of fear may be affected. So here are parts of the brain affected by anxiety. (I. Martin, J. Ressler, Binder & B. Nemeroff, 2013)[2]

Amygdala (It stores memories of emotional experiences and frightening events that occurred in our life.) People with anxiety have extremely sensitive amygdala. It will also react to non-threatening situations for them.

Hippocampus (It has the main role in processing emotions. It also deals with long term memories.) Hippocampus is also smaller in depressed people.

Locus Ceruleus (It determines which brain stimuli are worthy of attention.)

The prefrontal cortex (It is the part of the brain involved in making decisions, passing judgments, and problem-solving.) It can turn down fear response and is responsible for storing memories of situations of overcoming any fear. These two factors are key to treatment of anxiety.

Ways to reduce stress

•Listening to music will help greatly in dealing with a stressful situation. It has the power to calm down your brain, so it is fresh and ready for tasks ahead. Listen to calming music in a stressful situation could lead to being more productive than before.

•Give yourself a pep talk. Be your own boss. Sometimes, your only option is to rely on yourself. Stand in front of the mirror and try talking to yourself. It may seem crazy to others, but it is a very good technique to improve your thinking and get a clear head. Don't worry about seeming crazy; you have to build a little resilience and care less about what others think. It can go a long way in building confidence and fighting off stress caused by behaviors and the opinions of others.

•Some people, when under stress, tend to stop eating while others eat a lot. Both extreme behaviors are very damaging to health and only tend to make our stress levels worse than before.

•When under stress, all you need is a bit of perspective. You must ring up the person who can put things into perspective for you and give you a gentle slap of reality. Sometimes that's all it takes for stress to subside.

•Laughter is truly the best medicine. Laughing off a stressful situation is often enough for us to get out of whatever had us down. Laughter releases endorphins that will lighten one's mood. Try to incorporate laughter into your daily life.

•Green tea has been advised to be taken when in a stressful situation. It truly has a calming effect, not to mention the healthy dose of antioxidants.

•Lack of sleep is a straight one-way ticket to stress. Regular lack of sleep has an alarming number of bad effects on your mind and body. So always make sure to get the recommended good eight hours or so of sleep in the most comfortable environment that you can make for yourself. Yes, naps are revolutionary but have you laid down in bed under the covers and had a good night of sleep? It is the most effective stress buster out there.

•Short breaths are a cause of stress while deep breaths will oxygenate your whole body. It will sharpen your focus as it clears your mind.

What you call an anxiety attack may build up slowly. It is the hugely crushing feeling of worry and fear. The feeling of distress only gets worse as the event that troubles you gets nearer.

Anxiety can lead to addictive behavior. For example, alcohol is a sedative, it helps slows the activity of the brain and in turn, we feel relaxed and calm. What it is, is not a solution to get out of feeling anxious. However, most people suffering from anxiety in a social situation tend to abuse alcohol to help them calm down and relax. If this goes on regularly, it can lead to alcohol addiction. Alcohol will end up doing more harm than good because chronic addiction to it must be treated first.

Anxiety is directly related to avoidance behavior. It could lead you to separate yourself from important tasks out of fear. You will tend to avoid situations that worsen anxiety symptoms and are a cause of triggering them. These situations could be your school, workplace, or even the company of some people. It can prove to be detrimental, not for you but also the people surrounding you.

As they say, "adventure is dangerous, but a routine is lethal." For someone living a monotonous life in the same routine, falling into depression is pretty easy. You have to shake things up and try not to stick to routine too much. Take a break from work. Go on vacation and spend quality time with your loved ones. Don't let your work rule you. Take it from wise old people. They always advise the young to make memories and not run after money. I think it is high time that we finally listen to them.

Chapter 2: Mindfulness: The Best Way To

Manage And Relieve Anger

"The best way to capture moments is to pay attention. This is how we cultivate mindfulness. Mindfulness means being awake. It means knowing what you are doing." ~Jon Kabat-Zinn

Jon Kabat-Zinn's quote beautifully describes mindfulness as a state of complete awareness. Let us elaborate that so you can understand mindfulness and why it is the best way to manage anger.

Understanding Mindfulness

Mindfulness simply means to be patiently, non-judgmentally, gently, and carefully aware of each moment as it passes. Instead of attaching negative or positive sentiments to a moment and the activities of that moment, you perceive the moment for what it is. This helps you stay fully aware and conscious of your present, something most of us habitually ignore.

Yes, ignoring your present is precisely what leads to anger followed by stress, anxiety, and then depression.

Ignoring your present or not being aware of it is what we commonly call 'forgetfulness' —the complete opposite of mindfulness. Besides causing a variety of problems, forgetfulness also leads to anger, resentment, stress, and anxiety. Are you wondering how? Let me tell you a personal story that will elaborate this point.

A few years ago, my partner and I got into a big fight. He said things he should not have said, things that greatly upset me. Instead of letting go of that negativity and talking it out with my partner, I held on to his words.

I started to dwell in the past that had already happened. Instead of moving on, I kept thinking of his hurtful words; this slowly built resentment and anger inside me. We did not talk about that issue for days and as is often the case with unresolved fights, the pain wilted into the past and things slowly got better between us. However, I did not feel happy or at peace whenever my partner was around. I became bitter and angry, and was always in search of opportunities to vent out my anger on him.

With time, my anger issues exacerbated and caused strains in my relationship with him. I used to shout at him, fight with him, and humiliate him. Although doing that should have made me feel better, it did not.

As my partner and I were going through this vicious cycle, I discovered mindfulness and realized it absence in my life had almost sabotaged my relationship. I started reading all the mindfulness material I could find and practicing the various mindfulness strategies, I read about.

Although it took a while for my emotions and feelings to stabilize, and some additional time for the wounds between my partner and I to heal, consistent practice of mindfulness yielded AMAZING results.

As my state of mindfulness improved, I started to live in the present and began discarding concerns and worries about the past or future. As I became less forgetful, I started to enjoy my present, which helped me easily manage my anger issues.

As you can see, forgetfulness never leads to or births anything good. In fact, it takes you miles away from the present, the moment you live in, and shuts you in a cocoon of sadness, anguish, and negativity.

On the other hand, the state of mindfulness helps you become better in every aspect of your life. Why mindfulness, you may wonder. Are there no other effective ways to manage anger? If you are like most people, this question may bother you as you read this book. Here is the answer.

Why Mindfulness Is The Best Approach To Anger Management

Mindfulness is arguably the most effective and best approaches to managing anger and all its innate problems such as anxiety, stress, depression, and other emotional issues because if we are being truthful, all other anger management strategies and techniques have mindfulness as part of their core DNA. Does this sound confusing? To explain this, let us examine a few of the popular techniques used to treat anger, stress, anxiety, and depression vis-à-vis mindfulness.

Meditation: Meditation is indeed a wonderful practice that helps you understand yourself deeply. Not only does it make you calm, it also helps you fight anxiety, stress, and anger issues like a pro. How does it do that?

Meditation seeks to help you become better by improving your state of mindfulness. As your state of awareness becomes better, it becomes easier to focus on things and explore them to understand their effect on you. This core element is what helps you understand your anger and purge it out of your system instead of holding on to it.

Breathing Techniques: Deep breathing techniques are often the go to ways to manage anger, stress, and anxiety issues. Deep breathing enhances your sense of awareness and as such, helps you become and remain calm.

When you take shallow breaths, you start becoming anxious; anxiety clouds your ability to think clearly. As opposed to this, deep breathing calms you and as you relax, you become aware of yourself and surroundings. Hence, mindfulness is as well at the core of deep breathing.

Journal Writing, Dancing, Coloring, and Doing Enjoyable Activities: All these strategies certainly help you relax, manage your anger, and reduce anxiousness. However, they too, employ mindfulness to help you achieve those results.

When you write in your journal, you become aware of the negative thoughts that instigate anger; this improves your state of mindfulness. When you dance to the tune of something enjoyable, color, draw, or do anything you enjoy you become fully and mindfully engaged in that activity.

As your involvement in an activity increases, you take interest in it and start to live in the present; you already know what this does: it enhances your state of mindfulness.

Positive Self-Talk: Practicing positive self-talk whenever you feel angry, agitated, or anxious is another potent way to manage your anger and this technique too, draws on mindfulness.

When you give yourself positive suggestions, you divert your attention away from everything that triggers your anger and upsets you, and instead focus on the happy things in life. As a result, you become more mindful of your present.

As you can see, every strategy or technique aimed at self-improvement or eliminating any sort of unconstructive and negative habit, thought, emotion, practice, or feeling from your body, mind, and life has an element of mindfulness. From this, it is safe to conclude that mindfulness is indeed the best all-round remedy for anger, stress, anxiety, and depression.

Now that you have enough understanding of mindfulness and its amazingness, move to the next chapter to get started with lots of mindfulness-based techniques you can use to manage your anger, let go of stress and anxiety, become happier, and more peaceful than ever.

Chapter 3: How Depression Is Diagnosed

"Early diagnosis is so important because the earlier a mental illness can be detected, diagnosed and treatment can begin, the better off that person can be for the rest of his or her life." (Rosalynn Carter)

When you or someone you love is exhibiting several of the symptoms that were explained in the previous chapter, it is recommended that he or she be brought to a psychologist or psychiatrist so that proper treatment can be administered.

The clinical depression cure is very commonly administered because of the persistently high rate of the disorder. Early detection and treatment result in a much better chance of treatment.

The first part of the treatment is to identify the signs and symptoms of depression so as to determine if the person is experiencing depressive illness or simply a bout of sadness. A psychologist or psychiatrist administers this diagnosis using a criteria based on the Diagnostic and Statistical Manual of Mental Disorders - 4th Edition (DSM-IV).

A physical examination is also conducted along with an evaluation of the person's family history, so as to narrow down the proper depression cure. The patient will be interviewed to trace the triggering factors and identify the onset of the depression. All the findings will then be discussed and medication will be prescribed.

The doctor will highly likely order the patient to undergo a series of lab tests as well, so that he or she can rule out any other illnesses that manifest symptoms similar to depression. These are: Complete Blood Count (CBC), Electrolytes, Thyroid function tests and Thyroid-stimulating Hormone (TSH) level, Serum Toxicology Screen (drug test), and BUN and creatinine (for kidney issues). Other possible tests that will be administered to the patient are the MRI, CT scan or Electrocardiogram

(ECG) to check for heart problems and the electroencephalogram (EEG) to check for brain problems (including epilepsy).

Additionally, psychometric tests are also administered to help determine the right depression cure. One is the Beck Depression Inventory or the BDI, which is used to check depression based on the criteria found in the DSM-IV. Another is the Zung Self-rating Depression Scale, which is a more detailed questionnaire that is used to test for affective, somatic and psychological symptoms of depression. Another test is the Criteria for Epidemiologic Studies-Depression (CES-D) scale, which is another guide in identifying symptoms.

Specific tests are also administered based on one's age. Older adults often undertake the Yesavage Geriatric Depression Scale, while children between 6 and 17 years old take the Children's Depression Inventory (CDI).

Once depression has been clearly identified and all other possibilities are eliminated, treatment can then commence. There are multiple options when it comes to a depression cure. The most effective one depends on the specific case of depressive illness that a person is experiencing. In the next chapter, you will be introduced to the different options.

Chapter 4: Aging Before Your Time

People have always said that there are young people with grown up attitudes and that there are those in their twenties and thirties who seem much older. One of the problems associated with aging is highlighted in a study by a team of researchers from Umea University (3), who studied the effect of stress and the role it plays in the lives of people who suffer depression. You may be totally unaware of this, but within your body are things called telomeres. A chromosome is indeed wrapped into a telomere that really coats the outer layer of the chromosome and come in different lengths.

The interesting part of this study was that shorter telomeres are actually associated with depression and – once again – the level of cortisol within the body. Thus, those with shorter telomeres were prone to age more rapidly than those with longer telomeres. The scientists did their study on 451 patients, 91 of whom were known to suffer depression and stress related disorders. Interestingly enough, those who suffered depression were shown to be people whose cortisol levels were not regulated in the same way as those who were non depressive or not stressed. Thus, it can be seen that people who are in situations of stress and who are prone to depression are more likely to age before their time due to the cortisol levels being irrational.

So how can you regulate the cortisol release?

Prevention.com (4) have come up with a very good way to control this release and you may be surprised that many of these ways involve relaxation and enjoyment. Thus the following exercises are ones that can help you to control and regulate cortisol release in balance with other hormones within your body.

• Listening to music

• Buddhist meditation

- Drinking black tea

- Getting a good night's sleep

- Learning about spirituality

- Enjoying yourself

While these sound fairly easy for people who have balanced lifestyles, they are not as simple as you think for people who are stressed. Let's take one of them at a time and show you how to incorporate this into your life to benefit your health. When listening to music, for example, many multi taskers are doing other things. It is better for you to immerse yourself into the music. Lie down, absorb the music and give yourself a set amount of time each day to do this. It could be when you come in from work, or it could be in the lunch hour of a particularly stressful day. If you can't get home to immerse yourself in music, go to the park, put on your earphones and close your eyes so that the level of absorption is the same. This way, you shut off the stress and are able to feed your mind with positivity, which strengthens your focus and sharpens your mind.

Buddhist Meditation

We hear often that Buddhist meditation is a good thing, though how good is it really? In 1992, Richard Davidson (5), of the Department of Psychology at the University of Wisconsin decided to do a study on positive emotions and was a little startled by receiving a fax from the Dalai Lama, offering to help. What he offered though was of interest to Davidson who took the opportunity to go to Tibet and perform tests on Buddhist monks. The full story may be of interest to readers, but what is more interesting is the results. The activity in the left prefrontal cortex, which is the area of the brain responsible for positive thought, in one particular monk, was higher than he had seen in all of his 175 subjects. Read this overview that came as a result of Davidson's studies and you will see why Buddhist meditation is relevant to stress.

"The "Monk experiments" at Madison are beginning to intersect with a handful of small but suggestive studies showing that Buddhist-style meditation may have not only emotional effects but also distinct physiological effects. That is, the power of meditation might be harnessed by non-Buddhists in a way that along with reducing stress and defusing negative emotion, improves things like immune function as well. "

This is a direct quote from the above research report that shows that the Buddhists may actually have got something right. Does that mean you have to wear saffron colored robes and sit and gaze into space? Of course not. Meditation in the manner of Buddhists can be achieved by putting several things into practice. Meditation is about concentrating on the breathing, but it's also about being aware and non-judgmental – in other words observing without getting emotionally involved with whatever is happening. It follows the rules of Buddhism, which were brought about, by the thoughts and philosophy of Gautama Buddha when he was trying to find out why humanity suffered so much. What he concluded was that mankind suffers because of the actions of human beings. Buddhism was created as a philosophy to correct that and to end the suffering of mankind.

Exercise in Buddhist meditation

For beginners, the best way to start meditation is to perform breathing meditation, which is when you are seated with your back straight in a comfortable position. Many will choose to sit on a cushion and bend the knees, crossing the ankles, though this isn't obligatory. You do need to find a place where you will not be disturbed, however, and wear comfortable clothing that does not constrict you in any way. Close your eyes and breathe in through the nostrils thinking of nothing except that breath as it comes into your body. Feel it going down into your upper diaphragm, hold the breath for a moment and then breathe out through the nostrils, concentrating only on the energy of that breath.

It's very hard to do at first because your mind, when you are stressed, is going to be filled to brimming with all kinds of thoughts. It's hard to ignore them since this is not what you are accustomed to doing. However, you need to persist. When you exhale count to one through to ten on each exhale and if you think about other things, go back to one again.

Some people do this in a calm natural environment but if you are new to this style of meditation, it may be a good idea to choose a nice quiet area near your pool or in your garden where no one will disturb you.

This kind of meditation sharpens the mind and makes you a lot happier in yourself. When you are stressed, you don't have the space to stop thinking unless you actually create that space. Give yourself a twenty minute session a day and you will feel the benefits of it fairly soon. Your subconscious is able to work on problems while you are busy relaxing! That's quite some feat but it's worth it because it helps you to feel happier about life and lowers your stress levels.

By lowering your stress levels, you are able to relax more and release valuable endorphins in your body that help you to feel better about life. These are the "feel good" hormones that are released by the brain which allow you a sense of wellbeing. Tom Scheve wrote a very good article (6) on endorphins that will explain to you the significance of them and what they do to the body. It is endorphins that give the body its natural high and these can be released during meditation just as they can be during enjoyable exercise.

If your stress levels are particularly high, then meditation is your friend. Once you learn to focus the mind on your breathing, you should think of it as a flow of energy rather than just air passing into your body. Follow the energy as you meditate. Feel it flow through you and the end result is that endorphins will be released which lesson your stress and make you feel much more at one with yourself and the world around you. Remember not to think of it in terms of breathing. Think of that breathing in terms of energy because that's what it is. It's your lifeblood and it's what makes you wake up every morning. It therefore deserves that respect.

Chapter 5: Affirmations And Self-Concept

Your self-concept is the master program of your internal computer. It works like your psychological operating system. Every thought, emotion, feeling, experience, and decision you've ever had is forever recorded on this psychological hard drive. Once recorded, these sensations then affect the way you feel, think and act from that moment onward.

Your self-concept predicts the levels of productivity in every part of your life. Your self-concept describes why the psychological laws have such an unreasonable effect on your individuality.

You have a self-concept for driving, a self-concept for dancing, a self-concept for work, a self-concept for romance, a self-concept for how much you eat, a self-concept for how much money you earn. To save some time, you hold a self-concept for every aspect of your life.

The moment your self-concept in a specific area is formed, you will act and think in a way uniform with it. This is a self-fulfilling prophecy, since if you think and act as you've always thought and acted, you will continue to think and act in this way.

Here's How to Break the Chain

Your self-concept is putting along, as it always does. That means you will come across situations that affirm your self-concept (all self-concepts justify themselves, or else they would self-destruct due to inconsistencies).

In these moments, you are given the opportunity to take a giant bat and swing it at the giant machinery that is your negative self-concepts.

For example, you go golfing, and you miss many swings. You slice and hook the ball into the tall grass, and you become very discourages.

You have two options in how you think;

1) first, you can think a negative thought: "I'm rubbish at golf, and I will never get good". OR

2) you pick a more positive thought: "I might just be having a bad day; nothing to worry about, as I'll stay persistent and improve over time"

Here's the secret to this; you only need to choose a thought that is the slightest bit more positive than how you're feeling at that moment.

In the same example, if your mind went to "I'm the worst player in golf!" after missing a stroke, you can improve on that by saying "Maybe I'm the second worst player in golf!". This is actually believable, so your mind won't reject it.

You can up the ante with further thoughts and affirmations that you believe. As you continue, your mood will lighten, and you can base yourself upon that and find thoughts that will actually put you in a better mood than you were originally:

"Maybe if I practice, tomorrow I'll be the third worst player in the world."

"I wonder who the number one worst player in the world really is.."

"Maybe he can give me golf lessons."

"Or better yet, we can hold a golf tournament between all the worst players, in which the highest score wins"

"What a holler that would be! They be aiming for birds (and missing, of course)"

Eventually, you can remove the negativity and soul-crushing self-identity:

"Oh, there's no point in being mad about my golf skills today! I'll just get through this and try to improve for the next time."

Always choose a better thought, and do this enough times, and your thoughts will become more positive. You can do this in every area of your life.

Of course, this takes work and consistency; after all, you are, in fact, upgrading your operating system (and consequently, your self-concept and confidence).

Doing this exercise ultimately will direct your feelings to a far better place. As you do this, you will gradually approach your self-concept to your self-ideal, and to match it in actual facts.

Your self-concept can be your very own self-ideal. This is often the ideal picture or image you hold in yourself. You can fantasize as though you're already the best version of yourself. Your self-concept and self-ideal is comprised of your hopes, wishes, goals, dreams, and fantasies about your suitable future life, together with the qualities and virtues that you appreciate most in yourself and in others. Your self-concept (if high) and self-ideal is a composite through favorable thinking of the best person you can imagine yourself being, living the best life you could live.

High performing, happy, successful people have very obvious and powerful self-ideals. They have clear ideas of whatever they'd like to have. They hold clear beliefs

51

about the values, virtues, and features of the superior women and men that they wish to emulate. The most successful individuals have an uplifting, inspiring concept of what an excellent person emanatesand how she or he behaves in their self-concept.

Here's an exercise: what exactly are the results that you would like to have in your everyday life? Which feelings do you think are connected with those results? Then, consider those thoughts as much as you possibly can, as they will program your mind towards achieving success in these areas.

Whatsoever your self-concept, your pattern of thinking (if left unchallenged) pertaining to money or other area of productivity, becomes your comfort-zone. After that point, your comfort-zone becomes your greatest obstacle to increased performance. After you get into a comfort-zone in every area, your subconscious strives and does its best to remain in the comfort zone, although it might be vastly below what you're really capable of accomplishing within that area.

The solution to achieving your fullest potential and cultivate the same habits of prosperous individuals would be to raise your self-concept in beneficial thinking ways. It's for you to cultivate new habits of constructive thinking regarding what is achievable for you. The manner in which you accomplish greatly more on the outside is simply by changing your feelings and thoughts about your possibilities in that area inside.

Chapter 6: How To Build Self Confidence

Through learning how to be confident and improving self-esteem, we can greatly enhance our lives. Confidence helps us to reach our goals, find success and achieve a greater over-all feeling of self worth. Information will form the foundation of your efforts to build self confidence.

Why is Confidence Building so Important?

Your level of self confidence can and usually will, have a very significant impact on your life. It is deeply intertwined in our psychology and affects nearly everything we do in some way. In addition, it greatly affects the way you view yourself, the way others view you, the relationships you form, the opportunities you get, the decisions you make and the actions you take throughout your life. This is one of the reasons why it is important to learn how to build confidence.

So now we know what it is, how can you build on it? Here are five ways that might help.

1. Smile

This might sound silly but you don't smile if you're feeling unhappy or nervous. The simple act of smiling, even if you have to force it at first, will make you feel better. A smile is something everyone associates with positive feelings, so by smiling you make yourself feel better, you will appear confident, other people will notice and they too will feel less nervous and more confident. Before you know it you will fit right into the situation that you were nervous or lacking in confidence about.

2. Good Posture

How you carry yourself tells a lot about you. If you slouch or walk around with your shoulders slumped forward with your head down, you don't give off any feelings of confidence to yourself or anyone else. So always stand up straight, with your head up and make eye contact with everyone you meet. This will make a positive impression on those you meet which will reflect back on you making you feel more confident.

3. Be Grateful

When you thing about what you want, your mind comes up with reasons why you can't have it e.g. you don't have the money, you don't deserve it, you don't need it. This leads you to think about lack and brings on more negative thinking which does nothing for self-confidence. The best thing to do is to focus on what you have and be grateful for it. It is something you should do daily and you should go through a list of things you are grateful for. Think about the friends you have, good things you have done in the past, any skills you may have, good relationships you have or had. This will bring about positive thoughts and when you are having predominantly positive thoughts you feel better, more motivated and definitely more self-confident.

4. Appearance

I don't know about you but I know when I'm wearing tatty old clothes (we've all got that part of jeans and shirt covered in paint with holes in that we use for odd jobs around the house) I don't feel that good. I look at myself and think 'you look a mess' and then I don't feel that great either.

Nothing beats getting out of the old clothes, having a shower and a shave and getting into something clean and tidy looking. The improvement to your confidence is amazing.

5. Say Something

Now strange as it may seem, if you are with a group of people you have just met, one of the best ways to help increase your confidence is actually to say something. You'llquite likely find that other people in the group are just as nervous about speaking as well. If you make the effort to speak, even once, within a group you'll become better at speaking in public and become more confident.

So there you have 5 pretty easy ways that you can use to help build up your self-confidence. As with all things it takes a bit of perseverance, but even if all you do is smile and stand up straight that is a good start to developing your confidence.

Chapter 7: Who Can Practice Meditation?

Children

There is a misconception that meditation is only for elders. This is not true. Even kids can practice meditation. Meditation can help a child understand themselves from an early age, and lead to a successful and fulfilled life. Meditation has even been found to help kids with ADHD and autism. Many of the problems that we face in life stem from insecurity. Psychologists are of the opinion that insecurity and unhappiness from an early age is what makes people to take on destructive lifestyles. Meditation can help combat these feelings early on, so that the rest of their life will be a bit easier to deal with. Childhood is the time that shapes your subconscious mind; it sets the standard that will continue for the rest of your life. In an ideal world, meditation would be taught to children in schools. After all today's children are the citizens of tomorrow.

Children are easily discouraged by lengthy sessions, and that is why almost all of the meditation courses offered to children are only for a day. There are several meditation techniques that you can choose from, but of all the techniques the best choice would be Anapanasati meditation. This is a mental purification process that is achieved by self-observation. Children are very observant, so this is the right time to mentally train your child. Anapanasati meditation involves the observation of your natural respiration, the inhalation and exhalation. This step can help your child in mind concentration. Aside from that, this technique can also quiet your child; help him/her to understand himself better and how his/her mind works. Your child can develop inner strength to help him/her in choosing the appropriate and right actions over the wrong ones. Anapanasati meditation can provide your child with the right tool to face up to anxieties, fears, and childhood pressures.

Teens/ Young Adults

"I split hairs as my daughter/ son is entering teens", is an oft repeated statement said in exasperation by parents around the globe. Teenage can be quite annoying for the parents as well as the teenager. There are physical changes happening in youngsters and the hormones surge making them behave irrationally. This may seem normal to the teenager but can be frustrating to the parents. Meditation can help teenagers' to focus on their education and not get diverted from what matters. Focusing the mind on issues like creative pursuits, career goals, and higher education can keep him/her away from unwanted temptations.

Adults

Meditation is the panacea to all adult problems. Better to relax and start a meditation practice. Guided meditation and mindfulness can help adults to free the mind from stress and worries. Whether you're a sportsman or a sales person, meditation will help you to stay focused and positive. There are powerful techniques like yoga nidra, anter maun, or inner silences that can help you to control emotions and keep calm. These techniques are discussed in detail in the next chapter.

Seniors

When you're in the twilight years of life with less to look forward to, meditation keeps you rooted. Seniors often dwell upon their past and blame themselves for certain mistakes. A session of meditation in the morning can keep the mind calm, quiet and positive. In fact evening meditation can help seniors to get sound sleep.

How to practice meditation?

Make it a daily routine

First and foremost don't think that meditation is an exercise that you've to practice daily. Think about it as a way of life. Just like you brush your teeth or drink juice, make meditation a daily routine. Meditation should be practiced on a daily basis yet you can see the results after a month or two. Don't expect instant results.

Indentify space

Choose a quiet corner in your home. If you live near the sea, a forest, or mountains, you can go out and practice there. Nature is the perfect place to meditate. In case you're using a room at home, keep the place neat and clean. Place some aromatic candles and fresh flowers in the room. Make it a haven where you can learn to love yourself. The room should be that special place where you leave behind all your worries and get enveloped with peace, love and lasting happiness.

Art of visualization

Visualize yourself to be a calm and quiet person and you'll soon see yourself becoming one. There have been many studies about the power of visualization. Athletes have been known to practice this as well.

Positive affirmations

To move out of the rut of negativity, you have to reprogram your mind. Develop awareness within yourself about your thoughts and keep a watch on them. Make a list of powerful, energizing, positive, and motivating words and revise it often to improve on it. You can even select a word for the day and do meditation on it. This will improve your style of talking by forming emphatic and dynamic sentences. This is how you improve your vocabulary of good, motivating, positive words. Once you have formed a word bank of these, you can go ahead and utilize them in your daily affirmations and they will work wonders for you!

Road blocks for meditation

•Pain

Pain in your legs and body is familiar, particularly while sitting in the pose in which is new to you. Instead of at once shifting when you feel discomfort, keep still and observe the pain and the feeling it invokes inside you. Visualize as if you are a third person observing yourself. Regular practice will reduce the pain and after a time you will get used to it.

Initially when you sit crossed legged for prolonged periods; you experience lack of sensation in the legs.

• Distraction and restlessness

The only solution is to not worry about your thoughts running helter-skelter, at first. Just relax. Even if you've observed it, ignore. Don't dwell on it. If you are trying to clear your mind and have thoughts constantly coming into your mind, don't get upset with yourself. It takes time to master this skill. Simply recognize that your mind is wandering, and push the thought from your mind. Over analyzing is the enemy here.

Benefits of meditation

If you're still not sold on the idea of meditation, have a look at this chart for a few more examples of the benefits, though the list goes even beyond this.

Physical Benefits

Mental BenefitsSpiritual Benefits

Relief from MigraineHelps in anger managementYou reach a higher plane of consciousness

Cures asthmaKeeps mind calm & composedYou can control your thoughts

Reduces blood pressureGives inner peaceYou're the master of your destiny

Purifies blood and keeps blood sugar under controlCombats stress & tensionYou've the power to make things happen in your life

Reduces painRadiates inner beauty

Controls shaking in Parkinson's patientsKeeps you happy

Cures stomach ache and acidityLearn to cope with tragedies and failures life throws at you

Chapter 8: Identify And Acknowledge

Your Fears

The very first step to solving a problem, sickness or menace is the identification of such. You cannot possibly proffer solutions to a problem you are in the dark about. Hence, if you must truly fight and overcome your fears, if indeed you seek freedom from the grim cage of fear and desire to explore and maximize your potentials then you must identify your fear and its peculiarities. Identifying your fear will afford you the opportunity to critically dissect the causes and the probable way to overcome it. What is keeping you from unleashing your talent and potentials? The society? Or are you just afraid to dare yourself? Identify what is impeding you, and orchestrate plausible strategies to overcome them.

3.1. Be Curious

"Curiosity will conquer fear even more than bravery will."-James Stephens

Being curious is one of the viable ways to identify and overcome your fears. Curiosity opens you up to many possibilities and bolsters your confidence. Fear closes up your imagination, divides your mind and the world, and places bars and barriers between other people and yourself. It shuts you away from the world. On the other hand, curiosity is full of excitement, enthusiasm and anticipation.Curiosity sharpens your view of things and gives you a different perspective and facilitates your understanding. Curiosity is habitual. You gain a mastery and control of your object of curiosity over time because it becomes natural and ordinary to you.

Here are few questions to help you identify and define your fear:

What is the foundation of your fear? Did it start with a negative experience? Is it related to some environmental factors at your childhood? For how long have you been plagued by this fear?

What thought lingers on your mind for longer than usual?

What topic makes you unnecessarily uncomfortable when mentioned or talked about?

What is the loftiest and hardest to achieve of your goals?

How does your fear affect you, your mood and your action? Do you avoid visiting your family in another state because you don't want to get on a plane? Does it cause you to stay in bed instead of getting up and going to a class you're afraid of failing? Figure out exactly what power your fear has over your attitude and mind.

Is the source of your fear really perilous? Fear can be a healthy emotion that protects us from harm by causing us to escape things that are detrimental. Determine whether you have a good reason to be afraid or if your fear is misplaced and inhibiting.

3.2. Acknowledge Your Fear

Having identified your fear, there is no glory or beauty in living in self-denial. The denial of it does not help you overcome it, rather it compounds and complicates it leaving you in disarray. It is almost seamless to pretend as if our fears are illusive in a society that pays so much attention to bravery and being strong at heart. However, courage is insignificant unless you have some fear to fight. A sincere acknowledgment of your identified fear is a bold step towards having control over your situation. The acknowledgment of your fears drives and propels you devise practical means to overcome it. It is vital that you tag your fear and write it down. Putting down your fear in ink and paper is a concrete step to admitting that there is a challenge you want to overcome. It is also necessary to keep a working journal to monitor your progress as in your bid to fight your fears, showing clearly what measures you have put in place and how effective or otherwise the measures are. This gives you a long lasting victory over your fears because handling it as something that has a beginning and an eventual end can assist you to gain power to curtail it.

Chapter 9: What Is Social Anxiety?

A person with social anxiety is equally anxious in social situations and in person too. The comfort and security of your home is not enough to end your anxiety. In fact it is a great place where you can mull over how you could have handled the situations differently or how people were watching you all the time when it happened. Even though you are out of the situation, you can still feel the extreme anxiety associated with it.

It almost rewinds the incident in your head and plays it over and over again. The more you play the awkward parts again, it gets stored more and more into your brain. This adds to the assumptions of fear and humiliation you might go through the next time you are in such a situation. As a result the person might completely drop out of any event in the future and prefer to stay at home mulling over a past incident.

Such people usually know that their fears are completely baseless but they feel helpless and fail to overcome their anxious thoughts. Sometimes, they may even go out of their way to completely extract themselves from an event.

People with anxiety disorders go through a barrage of anxious thoughts which include:

•Thinking of all sorts of embarrassing situations they can get into.

•Completely avoiding speaking during an event fearing humiliation.

•Feelings of regret over how they could have handled the situation differently and how they fail every time.

Social Anxiety soon becomes a full-blown problem and makes us tremble or shake every time we are in a public situation. There are 3 tips given below that can help to you ease your anxiety.

1)Watch your feelings: Take a moment and try to notice how you feel when you get anxious.While you are busy worrying about what would happen next, do you light that cigarette or sip on your espresso?Rather than resorting to such unhealthy methods which only aggravate the problem, try meditation or deep breathing. As per research, people who use meditation techniques are better equipped to cope with their anxiety issues.

2)Watch your thoughts: When you are all set to give that job interview, do you think you are not good enough? Or that you may not get the job? Ask yourself what's the worst that could happen? Chances are, just like you thought, you won't get the job. But that is not the only job in the world. There are thousands of opportunities where you can test your skills. It is always better to get a job where you can make optimum use of your talents.

3) Watch what you do: Avoiding situations due to anxiety is a habit that a socially anxious person develops. But escapism does not lead you anywhere. So, the moment you feel tempted to opt out of a

situation rather than facing it, think of it as an ideal opportunity to end your issues and go for it. Human beings need to be in each other's company to lead a sane life. When you open yourselves to different situations, it gives you a chance to interact with people from various backgrounds. This can have a positive effect on the way you think.

Quick Facts - Did You Know?

•Social Anxiety Disorder is highly prevalent in our society and yet a much neglected disorder. It is the 3rd most chronic mental disorder in the U.S. affecting about 36% of its total population.

•Anxiety disorder is curable if diagnosed early, but unfortunately one-third of those suffering, receive treatment.

•People with social anxiety 3 to 5 times more likely to consult the doctor and about 6 times more likely to be hospitalized for psychiatric disorders

•Early signs of the disorder can also be witnessed in children in the form of excessive crying

Chapter 10: Triggers

At the age of 14, he had lost his mother to cancer.She had suffered for 2 years with the debilitating disease until finally, her body gave in and her spirit gave up.He was angry, he was hurt, and he had no coping skills whatsoever to deal with the loss.A year later, he left home, joined the military and put all of his focus and energies into his military career.He suppressed his mourning instincts, choosing instead to self-medicate and it worked.For a while.Anytime the term "cancer" was mentioned, he began to sweat, his heart raced and he was at the verge of panic. It was not until he turned 50 that he realized what was going on in his head, so he sought help.

There are positive memories and negative memories stored in the fascinating thing called the human mind.Tucked away we have memories of our first love, our first kiss, our first piece of pie, our first dance, or our first experience with social media.Many of those trigger feelings of joy, the brain releasing endorphins and the pleasure center of the brain is stimulated and it overwhelms the very existence of our being.

Conversely, there are terrible experiences that our mind often stores in much the same way.Hurts, losses, disappointments, and frustrations all exist in the same neurological store room as our joys.The problem is that for many people, the circumstances of events around is "trigger" the negative more often than they do the positive.

The second step in handling anxiety and panic attacks is to understand your triggers, identify what circumstances bring about the attacks of anxiety or panic.

These triggers could include:

•Memory of a loss (see above).

•Fear of rejection (social phobia).

•Nothing at all (arbitrary moments of anxiety with no reason).

•Unrealistic expectations (for yourself and by others).

There are a plethora of reasons why anxiety or panic attacks may manifest themselves and it is truly up to you to determine what they are.One specific recommendation is to:

Write It Down:As crass and blasé as it may sound, taking copious notes about the circumstances surrounding the anxiety occurance or the panic attack will serve you in the long and short-term.Ask yourself the following questions every time they occur:

1.What is happening right now?

2. What am I feeling physically and emotionally?

3. Leading up to the moment of anxiety, what was happening - what were you doing?

4. What did you have to eat that day for breakfast, lunch, and dinner?

5. What was/is your caffeine consumption?

6. Did you have any contact with anyone at the time of anxiety?

These questions will give you a safe and sound boilerplate to determine for yourself what the causal factors are to your anxiety and panic attacks.As the attacks or bouts of anxiety come or go, you'll see a pattern, perhaps.A series of events that led up to the moment when the anxiety hit.The people around you, the internal stimuli, the emotional influencers, your diet, and even caffeine intakecan greatly contribute to moments of extreme duress.

First, you understand and accept the fact that you're not alone.Secondly, you learn your triggers, the circumstances that facilitate your panic attack.

In the next chapter, we're going to take a hard look at some of the alternatives to pharmaceuticals that can assist in bringing

your anxiety and panic attacks under some
sense of control.

Chapter 11: Major Treatments For

Anxiety Disorders And Phobias

The major aim of most treatments for treating anxiety disorders and phobias is to help you reduce the symptoms so that the anxiety disorder and its attendant effects can no longer affect your everyday life. These treatments may include one or more of the following:

NON-Medication TREATMENTS

•Understanding

Understanding the cause of the symptoms, and talking things over with a friend, family member or health practitioner may help. In particular, most people worry that most physical symptoms of anxiety, such as palpitations, are due to a physical ailment. This can make the anxiety worse. Understanding the fact that you have a serious anxiety disorder is not enough to get you cured, but it will go a long way to help you on the journey to getting over the problem.

•Counseling

This may help some people with certain types of anxiety disorders. For instance, counseling which focuses on problem-solving skills may give some kind of help to people suffering generalized anxiety disorder.

Anxiety Management Courses

These maybe an option for certain conditions, if courses are offered in your area. The courses may include: problem-solving skills, learning how to relax, coping strategies, and group support.

Cognitive and behavioral therapy

The therapies, if available in your area, can work well for persisting anxiety disorders and phobias:

•Cognitive therapy is based on the notion that certain thought patterns can fuel, or trigger, certain mental health problems such as depression and anxiety. Your therapist helps you to understand your present thought patterns-most importantly, to identify any unhelpful, harmful, and false notions, beliefs, or thoughts you may have that can likely result in anxiety or depression.

•The major aim is then to change you thought pattern in order to avoid these ideas. Also, to help make your thought pattern more helpful and realistic. Therapy is mostly done in weekly sessions of about 50 minutes each, for a couple of weeks. You have to participate very actively, and get homework in-between sessions. For instance, you may be asked to make a diary of your thoughts which occur when you get anxious or develop some physical symptoms of anxiety.

•Behavioral therapy aims at changing any behaviors which are considered either unhelpful or harmful. For instance, with phobias your behaviors or response to feared object is harmful, and the therapist aims to help you change this. Various techniques are used, depending on the conditions and circumstances. Several sessions are also required for a course of therapy just like we saw in the cognitive therapy.

•Cognitive behavioral therapy is a blend of the two where you stand to benefit from changing both thoughts and behaviors. Both cognitive and behavioral therapies do not look into past events; rather, they aim at or try to change your present thought patterns and/or behaviors.

•Self-help

There are several national groups that offer quality information, support and advice. These groups, your doctor or a practicing nurse, may help connect you to some local groups for face-to-face support. You can equally get leaflets, books, tapes and videos on combating stress and relaxation. They teach very simple but effective deep-breathing techniques and several other measures to relieve stress, help you relax better, and possibly get rid of your anxiety symptoms.

Medication

Antidepressant medicines

These are commonly used for treating depression, but also help you reduce the symptoms of anxiety even when you are not depressed. They work by interfering with your brain chemicals known as the neurotransmitters such as serotonin which may be one of the causes of anxiety disorders.

•Antidepressants do not work immediately. It takes about 2-4 weeks before their effects can be felt and the anxiety symptoms begin to give way. One common problem is that most people stop the medication after one week or more because they feel it is not helping them at all. This is often too soon to measure the effect of the medication on the condition.

•Antidepressants are not really tranquilizers, and are not usually addictive.

•Several types of antidepressants exist, each comes with its various pros and cons. Most differ in their possible side-effects.

However, selective serotonin reuptake inhibitor antidepressants are the most commonly used for anxiety disorders.

•NB: after some people with anxiety problems start taking some antidepressants, the symptoms of the anxiety disorder may get worse for some days before they start noticing some improvements. Your doctor or nurse may want to keep you under check in the first few weeks to know if you have any kind of problems.

Benzodiazepines

Benzodiazepines like diazepam was once the most commonly prescribed medication for anxiety. They were often regarded as the minor tranquilizers but they do come with some serious known side-effects. They are often very effective for easing symptoms of anxiety. The major problem is that they can be very addictive and can easily lose their effect on your anxiety symptoms if you keep taking them for over a few week. They can equally make you drowsy. They are no longer used much for persistentanxiety conditions and short-term, or once in awhile to help you get over some very bad spell if you suffer from persistent anxiety symptoms.

Buspirone

Buspirone is sometimes included in the prescription for the treatment of general anxiety disorder. Though it is not yet clear how this medicine works, it is known to be an active anti-depressant medicine. It is not addictive and is believed to affect the production and circulation of serotonin in the brain. Serotonin is suspected to be involved in causing anxiety symptoms.

Beta-blocker medicines

A beta-blocker such as propranolol, can help ease some of these physical symptoms like trembling, heart thumping, etc. They may not have a direct effect of the mental symptoms like worry.

However, some people find it easier to relax if their physical symptoms are eased. This works better in short-lived severe anxiety disorder. For instance, if you get more anxious before you begin your performance in a concert then a beta-blocker may help you ease the tension and anxiety.

In some cases, a combination of treatments like antidepressants and cognitive therapy may work better than using only one of the treatments.

Alcohol and anxiety.

Though alcohol has been found to ease the symptoms for a short period, don't make the mistake of believing you can cure your anxiety by drinking alcohol. In the long run, drinking alcohol cannot cure anxiety disorders. Drinking alcohol often to calm jumbled nerves can result in problem drinking and may make the anxiety and depression problems worse in the long run. If you are taking alcohol or some street drugs to ease anxiety, you need to see a doctor as soon as possible before things get worse.

Chapter 12: How Meditation Helps

Depression

Many people have heard that meditation will help depression, but most people are unable to grasp how meditation helps. This chapter is dedicated into helping you to understand how meditation will help you to battle depression, stress, and anxiety. No matter if it's mild anxiety all the way up to anxiety disorders that are harder to conquer. More and more people are suffering from depression due to daily experiences because people are not forcing themselves to understand why they feel something, confront their feelings, or grow as a person.

Some people do have legitimate reasons to feel depressed due to their situation, but no matter what, if you feel depressed, then it is something that you need to take into your own hands to fix. Even if you are already taking antidepressants, going to counseling, or using another method to help you with your depression, meditation can be added to any routine to help you get the desired results.

It Develops the Hippocampus

The hippocampus is the center of emotions, memory, and nervous system. Those who practice meditation are known to have a stronger hippocampus than those that suffer from depression, which often deal with a weaker one. This is not a change that will happen overnight or even in the first week that you're practicing your meditation, but it will strengthen your hippocampus over time.

This will help you to be a healthier and happier you. You will not likely notice these changes at first because it is a gradual shift in your emotions. A strengthened memory will help you to put events into perspective a lot easier as well, which will help to make sure that you do not overreact to events or occurrences as much, which can happen to those who suffer from depression.

It Develops Your Prefrontal Cortex:

The left prefrontal cortex, which is the part of your brain that controls happiness, was found to be very highly developed in meditation practitioners, as well as very underdeveloped in those diagnosed with depression. Your ability to find happiness will be determined by your ability to process information and put it into proper prospective. This requires a level of focus and mental awareness that meditation can give you. Happiness is extremely hard to come by when you're depressed. Even if positive events are happening to you. A developed prefrontal cortex will help you to see the happier events and interactions in life.

It Raises Your Serotonin Levels:

Meditation has been found to raise the levels of serotonin and norepinephrine, the same chemicals that are raised by anti-depressants. This doesn't mean that if you're on anti-depressants that you should quit them. Though, overtime you may not need them. Talk to your doctor as you get healthier to decide if you should cut down or cut them out altogether. Raising your serotonin levels naturally is incredibly healthy, and it does not have negative consequences. If you notice that meditation is making you extremely happy, then you'll want to add it more often. Even if you aren't noticing a difference, there is one that will build up over time, and you should stick with it.

A Feeling of Wellness:

Many people diagnosed with depression say it comes with a feeling of something missing, while meditation practitioners tend to feel that their lives are more whole. This is a general feeling of wellness that will help to make you feel more fulfilled. It'll help you to handle the boredom of daily tasks without feeling like they are pointless, which is a common trait for people who are depressed.

Meditation recreates the brainwaves that are used to treat patients with depression. Inner peace is one of the main reasons that people practice meditation, and you can find a spiritual peace in meditation as well if you choose to do so for spiritual meaning. It all depends on what you're looking for. Just go into a meditation session with your intent held clearly in your mind.

Chapter 13: Mindfulness

Techniques/Exercises

To start living a mindful life, it is critical to use some effective exercises that will help tame your thoughts so that you can start living in the present. Here are some mindfulness exercises that you can try.

Exercise 1: One Minute of Mindfulness

Step 1: Check your watch and note the time.

Step 2: Leave your eyes open.

Step 3: Focus all your attention in breathing. Feel your breath as it goes in and out. Be ready to catch your mind from wandering off. Return your attention to your breath when it does so.

Step 4: Do this for 60 seconds

Over time, you can gradually extend the duration. This exercise is a correct foundation of mindfulness meditation technique.

Exercise 2: Conscious Observation

Step 1: Pick an object lying around you.

Step 2; Hold it in your hand and let your attention to be fully absorbed in the object.

Step 3: Observe it for what it is, without assessment or intellectual studying.

Step 4: Notice how your mind releases thoughts of the past or the future and how different it feels to be in the moment.

Exercise 3: Listen to Music

Step 1: Obtain a source of music.

Step 2: Select the music that soothes you.

Step 3: Turn on the music.

Step 4: Focus on the sound and vibration of each note.

Step 5: Notice the feeling that the music brings within you.

Step 6: Appreciate thoughts that creep into your head and bring yourself back to the music and the current moment.

Exercise 4:Observing your Thoughts

Step 1: Sit back, close your eyes, and keenly observe your thoughts without judging them. Don't be involved in them.

As you go through this exercise, you will realize that your mind is quieting and the thoughts are becoming less stressful.

Exercise 5: The Eating Meditation

Step 1: Look at the food carefully.

Step 2: Smell it.

Step 3: Feel the texture in your mouth with the first bite.

Step 4: Take your time to feel the taste on your tongue.

Step 5: Do this for the next bite.

Step 6: Always do this for the first two bites of any food you take.

Exercise 6: Listening Mindfully

Step 1: Sit still.

Step 2: Listen to the many tunes around you.

Step 3: Tune out each one of them until you remain with one.

Step 4: Concentrate on this very one. It could be trees rustling.

Step 5: Just let the sound to flow over you and for you to flow into the sound without judging it.

Exercise 7: Mindful Showering

Step 1: Step under a running shower.

Step 2: Feel it as the water hits your head.

Step 3: Concentrate as the water flows down the rest of your body.

Step 4: In case your mind wanders off, appreciate the thoughts and bring your mind back without judging yourself.

Step 5: Let the peace in the flow of the water flow inside and outside you.

Exercise 8: Candle Meditation

Step 1: Light a candle in a darkened room.

Step 2: Sit down, not too close to the candle.

Step 3: Observe the flame of the candle.

Step 4: Do not think about anything.

Exercise 9: Mindful Speech

Step 1: Listen attentively to the person you are conversing with.

Step 2: Break for a second before you speak.

Step 3: Understand in your mind what your partner is talking about.

Step 4: Think of your reply and its impact before replying.

Step 5: Speak more calmly and slowly to infuse more peaceful content into the conversation.

Exercise 10: Mindful Hands Awareness Exercise

Step 1: Grasp your hands tightly.

Step 2: Hold for about 5 to 10 seconds.

Step 3: Release your hands.

Step 4: Focus your attention on the feeling for as long as possible.

Exercise 11: Tactile Exercise

This exercise can tell you how your body deals with discomfort and how your emotions rise.

Step 1: Pinch your arm.

Step 2: Focus on how it feels.

Step 3: Notice how the pain radiates out from the site where you pinch.

Step 4: Pay close attention on the emotion that it creates within you.

Exercise 12: Body Scan Mindfulness

Step 1:Lie down comfortably and loosen any tight clothing.

Step 2: Pay physical attention to the physical feelings and sensations of your feet then slowly let your awareness drift further up your body.

Step 3: Do the same gentle noticing for all your body parts.

Step 4: Drift your awareness gently back noticing any other part with discomfort, pain, and tension until your awareness settles back to your feet.

Exercise 12: Mindfulness Of Physical Discomfort

Step 1: Bring your awareness and attention to your breath

Step 2: Notice with gentle curiosity the physical sensation of taking in air and taking it out. Do this for 2 minutes.

Step 3: Focus your awareness on physical body on what feels uncomfortable and what feels comfortable.

Step 4: Narrow down your focus to especially the parts of your body that felt uncomfortable. Allow your awareness to sit with it but don't act on it.

Step 5: Notice the feelings and sensations in your body. Notice how they shift and change.

Step 6: Allow your mind to drift again to discover another place with discomfort.

Step 7: Repeat step 4

Step 8: Bring back your awareness to your breathing and notice each breath as you inhale.

Exercise 13: Empty Bowl Meditation

Step 1: Sit quietly and comfortably with your palms open and up, placed on your knees.

Step 2: Open your mouth and touch the tongue to the roof of the mouth behind the front teeth.

Step 3: Breathe comfortably paying attention to your breath as you inhale and exhale

Step 4: Picture yourself entering into your nose, sit in your nostrils and watch your own breath as it goes in and comes out.

Step 5: After a few minutes, go with the breath from the nostril deep down behind the navel where it stops. Stay there for a moment

Step 6: Follow the breath out during exhalation and stop at 10 centimeters in front of the nose.

The two stops are important because when your breath stops, your mind stops. It means that you simply exist without the body, breath, and mind, just like an empty bowl. You will experience present moment stillness surrounded by tranquility and peace.

The techniques we've talked about will only help you to be mindful when you want. But the problem with this is that we are always on autopilot, which means that the likelihood of you "wanting" to be mindful is pretty slim given our hectic life. This means that you ought to figure out a way of cultivating a habit of mindfulness. We will learn how to dot that in the next chapter.

Chapter 14: How To Be More Confident

When Socializing In A Group

In this chapter, we will see how you can become more confident when you're out with a group of people. They could be your friends, colleagues, clients, business partners, relatives, or just about any group of people that you happen to hang out with.

Introverts have some exceptional skills that are common to each one of us. If used in the right way, these skills can become our strengths. Let's see what these skills are and how they can help us become more confident when we are socializing.

Take advantage of your listening skills

Usually, introverts prefer to keep quiet and talk only when they have something valuable to add to the ongoing conversation. Sometimes, you do not talk even when you have something to say.

This is especially true when you are with people who you are not very close to.

This trait of introverts has naturally made them extraordinary listeners, a very rare, yet one of the most sought-after human qualities. Humans love talking and even when we pretend to listen, we are just trying to think of what we'll say next.

When the world is busy talking, introverts listen. They are capable of listening and understanding the things that others might miss.

Next time you are having a discussion in a social setting and you are able to spot something that no one else had noticed, then do share it with the group. You might have some really interesting insightthat wouldn't have been brought up otherwise.

People love it when you genuinely listen to what they have to say and they will admire you for this amazing quality.

Use your thinking abilities

This point is closely related to the last one about listening. Introverts are thinkers, in addition to being listeners. That is a fantastic combination. Introverts think all the time, so much so that it wouldn't be wrong to call some of themover-thinkers. But that's just how we are.

Can we use our thinking capacity to get us to talk? Of course! If someone proposes a solution or points at a problem, you could use your ability to think and analyze to quickly come up with rough inferences or even estimates.

For example, if someone in an office meeting says that our revenue has taken a hit in the past quarter, you could quickly think about the things that didn't quite work well for your organization or the changes that were brought about in the last quarter.

While you cannot be 100% sure, you can certainly give some of the possible reasons for the dip in revenue even before someone has actually sat down to analyze them. You can get people to think over the points raised by you.

This is an example of an office meeting, but the concept could be applied anywhere, even in your own personal social meetings. So, the next time you are out there socializing, do not hesitate to share your thoughts with the world.

You have some amazing ideas and the world needs to know them.

Break down the group into individuals

Picture this: you find yourself hanging out with the same group of people from work. While everyone in the group is quite comfortable with each other by now, you still find yourself being anxious when you have to go out with them every time.

It is true that introverts need more time than others to bond with people, especially if it's a group of people you have to bond with. It could be a bit overwhelming for you, but you know what? There is a way around this.

Instead of bonding with the entire group, try bonding individually, with each member of the group. It would be a lot easier for you to approach one person at a time and to get to know them better individually, rather than getting to know the whole group at once.

With time, you will be comfortable with every person in the group and eventually start having fun when you go out as a group.

Chapter 15: Prioritize By Organizing The

Essentials

We all know the importance of to-do lists. But the problem with most of these is that they are cluttered. This is where priority lists come in. They show a limited number of activities that are most important. Ideally, this list should only have 2–4 items.

It is argued that the mind can only focus on 3–4 things at a time. Any more than this stresses it. And lots of studies show that long to do lists are really a sure-fire way to stress your mind.

So I recommend having a priority list and not just a simple schedule. If you find you can't trim your list, then automate some tasks. If you cannot automate, then hire others to help you. Of course, you will first need to ensure that the tasks are only essential ones. Otherwise, follow the guide on setting goals.

Also, you must ensure that you keep your tasks on a single sheet of paper. This will make accessing them less taxing for your brain. And having a paper means you don't have to remember that you have a priority list somewhere – a paper can be kept beside your desk. No need to open applications, input passwords, etc.

Having Goals and Strategies

Most of the times, people fail to achieve dreams because of lack of clarity. So before you start decluttering your soul, you must have goals as well as strategies to guide you. These will set you on the right path if you go astray. And they will direct you on what to do in different situations. Blindly following your instincts may not be such a good idea.

For goals to be effective, they must adhere to certain principles:

Specific – don't just say I would like to declutter my life. Say the part of your life you would like to declutter. Do you have lots of useless goals? Do you have lots of negative feelings weighing you down?

Measurable – you need to know the progress you are making in following your goals. This means they must be set in a way you can easily measure. Of course, this can be easy or difficult depending on the goal in question. For things like schedules, it is easy since you just need to look at how many items you have on it. But for issues like feelings, it may be tricky sometimes.

Timed – you must set a limit by which the goal must be achieved. For example, you might say, "2 weeks from now, I will develop a habit of having a schedule with a maximum of 3 items."

Each goal you set must be accompanied by strategies. These will detail how you will achieve the goal in question. For example, if you are going to get rid of toxic relationships, how are you going to do that? Will you write emails telling the people concerned that you will no longer be seeing them? Or will you just start avoiding them?

Chapter 16: Habits

We are creatures of habit. Having a routine allows us to go through the day. Another option would be to think everything through and that would be a slow and exhausting process. Imagine if you had to think about everything you are going to do like, for instance, waking up and taking a moment to think which leg first you should step from the bed.

Habits are helpful but if we build bad habits they keep us in a downward spiral.

You will have to step outside your comfort zone and change your habits that have been ruining your health and had a negative effect on your mental state. Adopting positive habits feels somewhat uncomfortable at first. This is completely natural. Your current habits took time to form so adopting new ones will take some time to stick as well.

4.1. EATING AND DRINKING HEALTHY

First habit you need to adopt is a healthy diet. Keep yourself hydrated by having a source of water handy at all times. Eating healthy is a hard habit to adopt but luckily we live in an age of Internet and it is full of great tasting healthy recipes which take up to half an hour to prepare.

You have plenty of responsibilities that demand a lot of energy and leave you very little time. Cooking meals can be a great way to unwind and preparing portions for two meals makes overall time spent on food preparation less than unfreezing and cooking out-of-the box food.

You can find instructions on what you should eat and drink in the previous chapter.

4.2. SMILING

Thich Nhat Hanh said about a smile "Because of your smile, you make life more beautiful." Smile as often as you can. Start your day by smiling into a mirror, smile while you brush your teeth. Tell yourself that this will be a great day. Do this even if you do not feel like it and it feels silly.

Our facial expressions depend on how we feel but it actually works other way around. Studies have shown that smiling releases serotonin - a neurotransmitter that produces feelings of happiness and well-being. It is like a circle of happiness. Smile and you feel happy, you feel happy and you smile.

You can alter the way you feel by putting on a big smile. This might feel a little bit silly but little bit of silliness is a good thing. Sometimes we get so preoccupied with tasks and issues that we loose all joy of life. Little bit of silliness will help you bring back some of the joy of life you used to have.

Sometimes we need a little bit of help to get us started. Try to visualize a happy memory or a funny moment from your favorite comedy. I love slapstick comedies so every time I have difficulty putting on a smile I remember funny moment from the

Police Squad! or any other silly Leslie Nielsen movie.

Smiling will bring many advantages to your life as this habit will change how you feel and how people perceive you. Mother Teresa noted the importance of a smile, "Let us always meet each other with smile, for the smile is the beginning of love."

Smiling makes you look more approachable, friendly, warm and sincere. Building relationships requires both parties to be ready to open up and to allow another person to share worries, joys and experiences. Smile is an invitation.

Adopting the habit of smiling will allow your current relationships to improve and to build new ones. A simple smile is a very important tool you have to use to improve how you feel and to improve your life.

4.3. SLEEPING

Sleep is a mystery. We know that it is vital to get enough of sleep but scientists still can not pin point the reason why. Good sleep routine is vital for the physical and mental health. English dramatist Thomas Dekker expressed the importance of smiling very precisely, "Sleep is the golden chain that ties health and our bodies."

We are all aware of the risks involved in drunk driving but some countries are expanding a list of risks that they are taking into account. Studies have proven beyond any reasonable doubt that drowsiness is as dangerous as being drunk. Sleepiness affects your ability to concentrate, slows your reaction time, affects your ability to process information and impairs your memory. Truck drivers are already legally required to stop and have a rest and with risks involved it is no wonder that police officers are now checking regular drivers for drowsiness as well.

Sleep or lack of it affects your health as it is essential to get enough of quality rest in order to have a strong immune system. Study after study has revealed that people who sleep poorly are at a greater risk of getting sick or developing other health issues. Lack of sleep is one of the factors negatively influencing anxiety levels and your ability to deal with stress.

Long commute, work and other obstacles can make getting enough of sleep a mission impossible. You may feel pressured to get 8 hours of sleep a night but good news is that this rule does not necessarily apply to you. The number of hours you need depends on many factors and you should not feel pressured to get those 8 hours. Most adults can get enough of rest with 6 hours of sleep.

You can implement few changes that will help you fall asleep faster and improve the quality of your sleep.

These few simple improvements to your daily routine will help you get the rest you need:

-Do not use any electronic devices at least 1 hour before going to bed. It is important to prime your body for sleep. Do not watch TV or use any mobile device at least an hour before going to bed. This includes ebook readers. Spend this hour prepping your body for sleep by reading a book while sipping a cup of herbal tea and working on this program.

-No food at least 2 hours before sleeping. Plan your day in such a way that the last meal of the day is not too late.

-Evening is time to get ready for sleep so avoid caffeine. Skip coffee or black tea during the dinner and drink water or fruit tea instead. Avoid juice as it has high sugar content. By drinking beverages containing caffeine you are making it harder for yourself to fall asleep and once you are asleep, caffeine tends to cause nightmares.

-Eliminate light sources from your bedroom. Make your bedroom as dark as you can during the night. Due to a large number of various devices modern home contain, your bedroom might look like Star Trek control panel at night. Cover all those flashing lights as well.

-Go to sleep at a consistent time. Always be in bed at the same time. Your body will go into a pattern and falling asleep will be automatic. You might be inclined to stay up late on weekends to catch up to the show you missed during the work week but you need to go to sleep and to wake up at the same time during the weekend as well.

-Exercise. Increased physical activity improves your mood, health and reduces your risk of developing insomnia.

-Spend five minutes right before going to sleep writing down your plan for tomorrow. Recent studies have shown that writing a to-do list will 'offload' thoughts about tasks that need to be done and this reduces worry and allows you to fall asleep faster.

You may be inclined to cut corners and use alcohol or sleeping pills. Damage alcohol causes to your anxiety is extensively covered in the previous chapter. To give you a quick recap, alcohol has a direct negative effect on your organs and your nervous system. Any short term relief you might feel at the time of the alcohol intake is short lived as it is quickly replaced by spike in anxiety.

Drinking alcohol to get good nights rest is like smoking few cigarettes to improve your performance during a marathon. Alcohol blocks REM sleep and affects normal production of chemicals in your body. You end up waking up without actually getting the necessary rest. You may think that you need to sleep longer but the real solution is the elimination of alcohol and the same amount or even less time of sleep will allow you to get the rest you were dreaming about for so long.

Imagine waking up full of energy and well rested. This reason alone is enough to quit drinking.

The use of sleeping pills is a sensitive subject and you may be using them right now. Mounting evidence suggests that sleeping pills are as damaging to your health as smoking a pack of cigarettes a day.

Sleeping pills are thought to cause drowsiness, delayed reaction times and impaired balance, which can lead users to fall and break their bones. Research has shown that the risk of a fracture is doubled in those who rely on the drugs to get a good night's sleep. A study published online in June 2015 by the American Journal of Public Health found that people prescribed sleeping pills were around twice as likely to be in car crashes as other people.

List of possible side effects is long and worrisome. Long term studies show that sleeping pills can increase heart attack risk by a whopping 50%. Nottingham University researchers found that common pills may also increase the risk of contracting pneumonia and dying from it.

You may be risking your health to gain very limited benefits. Review of one of the leading over-the-counter brand of sleeping aid effectiveness has revealed that people who took a sleeping pill every night for three months fell asleep just 6 minutes faster on average than those who took a placebo. And those who used sleeping aid slept on average only 16 minutes longer than people given a placebo.

If you rely on sleeping pills right now be aware of the risks involved. Employ tactics we discussed above and hopefully soon you will be able to sleep without the chemical assistance. Used on a short-term basis, with the guidance of a physician, sleeping aids can help to break the difficult and often intractable cycle of insomnia and help get sleep back on track. However, the best long-term strategy is to develop a strong, sustainable sleep routine that does not rely on prescription sleep medication. There is no question this takes work, but the rewards are worth it. Your sleep, your overall health will be better for it.

4.4. EXERCISE

Development of anxiety disorders is closely connected to low levels of physical activity. It is extremely luring to fall into a daily routine. You wake up, go to work, come back home, watch some TV or play games and go to sleep. You feel exhausted and doing exercises seems like an impossible task.

A huge hurdle is a perceived lack of time. For most of us days are so crammed that the only option is either to do sports or to get some sleep. This is a problem that solves itself but you have to overcome initial resistance. All these habits require you to keep track of your days and to change what you consume, how you spend your days, evenings and nights.

Exercise is a powerful tool to improve your physical and mental health. All of these healthy habits are beneficial but you will feel significant results only if you employ all of them. Healthy habits multiply positive effects of each other.

Healthy eating and sleeping habits boost your energy levels and this gives you additional energy to exercise. Exercising improves your sleep and your health and this in turn allows you to reach for new challenges in your exercising routine and so on. This is the amplifying effect in action.

Exercise does not mean that you have to spend at least 1 hour at the gym each day and get a six-pack. Exercising means increasing your physical activity in your day-to-day life. You may not have possibility to spend time and money on a gym but tweaks to your daily routine will add up to produce amazing results.

Solution to the lack of time for exercise is replacement of current activities. Instead of watching TV, relax by going for a walk or a run. During your lunch brake you can go outside and eat your lunch outside. Any time you have left - spend it by walking few times around the block.

This simple change in your routine will work wonders. You will return to work refreshed and full of energy to finish tasks instead of just coasting for the rest of the day. Sometimes we get caught up thinking about obstacles and fail to notice solutions that are right in front of us.

Making this change has greatly improved my life and I implore you to do it. I used to eat my lunch either at my desk or in our break-room. I was able to tackle tasks for the first half of the day but after lunch I would feel as if my head was an empty box. Spending some time outside and that small exercise is like pressing a restart button.

It is as important to rest as it is to work. Exercising and being outside allows you to get necessary rest from your work and allows you to tackle tasks much more efficiently. This will reduce stress and overwork as your tasks will be finished on time and you will not have to fix mistakes.

Working while you are tired can be worse than doing nothing. You are much more prone to making mistakes which require you to review and fix everything again later. This way exercise and rest save you time.

Not getting enough of exercise hurts your immune system by reducing your ability to fight infections. Exercise causes changes in antibodies and white blood cells (WBC). WBCs are the body's immune system cells that fight disease. These antibodies or WBCs circulate more rapidly, so they could detect illnesses earlier than they might have before.

Finally, exercise slows down the release of stress hormones. Stress increases your chance of becoming ill and it has direct influence on your anxiety level. In his biography Arnold Schwarzeneggerexpressed this very precisely, "Training gives us an outlet for suppressed energies created by stress and thus tones the spirit just as exercise conditions the body."

You do not need to start lifting weights or running marathons. Being overzealous with exercise can be damaging if you are just starting out. Simply walk everywhere, take the stairs and use any opportunity to be physically active.

The best thing you can do is to join a team. It can be basketball, badminton or any other team sport. Being a member of the team will allow you to get mutual support, spend great time with new friends and it will be harder for you to quit as you will be committed to the team.

4.5. QUIT SMOKING

Smoking is nowhere near as common as it used to be just a few years ago but if you are one of the last ones to rely on cigarette to fight anxiety listen up.

For the sake of your health you have to quit.

Studies have unambiguously debunked myth that smoking reduces anxiety. Research has proven beyond any doubt that the opposite is true. Cigarette companies decided to tackle public health concerns by introducing other products like e-cigarette.

Anything with nicotine in it has a strong negative effect on you. E-cigarettes and similar products have been introduced with slogans that these are safe alternatives to regular cigarettes. Studies take time and now that the results are starting to come in it looks like e-cigarette is safer than regular cigarette but it still poses many long term health risks.

Nicotine by itself is a very nasty thing and you should not rely on it to reduce your anxiety.

Nicotine is a highly addictive chemical which affects nervous system and has a negative effect on your anxiety level. There are three main mechanisms how nicotine affects your mental state.

First, the ritual of smoking may feel like it reduces your stress and anxiety but calming effect is short-lived. Nicotine has a very short half-life. You feel the urge to smoke because you experience withdrawal symptoms. This makes you feel additional anxiety multiple times a day and this adds to your overall level of anxiety and stress. You are trying to fight fire by pouring gasoline on it.

Second reason is a failure to cope with anxiety on your own. Smoking essentially replaces your own natural ability to cope.

Stress coping is a mental skill, when you do not use it, you lose it. Smoking temporarily numbs anxiety but it does not actually help you cope, so your ability to cope with stress without the use of nicotine deteriorates.

This is the main reason most smokers fail to quit. Relying on smoking to cope with stress means that you loose your ability to deal with even a minor amount of stress without it. Smoking restrictions are constantly being expanded so an ability to cope with anxiety without the assistance of nicotine is essential skill you need to posses.

Finally, smoking exposes you to a huge number of dangerous chemicals. Healthy lifestyle is simply incompatible with smoking as cigarette smoke contains huge variety of cancerogens, poison and trash. Smoking or using other nicotine sources feeds addiction that ruins your health.

Smoking has the same effect on your body as experiencing stress. Your heart rate increases, your blood pressure shoots up and this closely resembles effects of stress. Your body feels these symptoms and it reacts accordingly.

Negative effects of smoking are well documented and are readily available to you in a huge number of reputable sources. You made excuses in the past but now you made a commitment.

If you want to eliminate panic attacks from your life and reduce anxiety to normal levels you have to quit smoking. There is no place for half-measures as all these changes will have significant effect only if you employ all of them.

Chapter 17: Meditation For Stress,

Anxiety And Depression

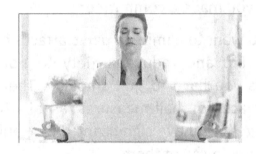

Regular meditation practice can benefit anyone, regardless of their physical or emotional health going into it. However, it is also worth mentioning that an overwhelming portion of the population suffers from stress, anxiety and depression even if they have never received an official medical diagnosis. The purpose of this book is to introduce you to the healing power of meditation, but it is especially important to bring light to the positive aspects of combining meditation with mental and emotional conditions such as stress, anxiety and depression. In this chapter we focus on meditation specifically for these emotional disorders that affect not only ourselves, but our loved ones, friends, neighbors and coworkers. Stress, anxiety and depression seem to be present on every corner of life. With meditation, we have the power to combat and beat these unwanted invaders of our time, energy and health.

Meditation and Stress

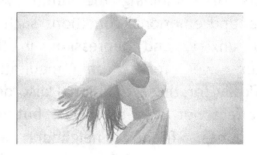

What do you think is the most common reason that people give for wanting to explore meditation? Most of the time the answer is "stress". Stress is an unavoidable fact of life. We feel it in different degrees throughout the seasons of life. Sometimes the stress is minor or self inflicted, while other times the stress is sourced from something serious and unavoidable. No matter the source, life will continue to present challenges, some of which have the potential to be stressful. The question is how can you best navigate these challenges and address stress in a healthy way rather than letting it eat away at your true happiness? This is what we know; we know stressful events are unavoidable, we know stress is individual and we might each experience it in a different way or at different degrees, we know that chronic stress is related to serious health consequences and we know that there is no magic pill to cure stress or prevent it from poking its head into your life. We also know that meditation can be a powerful tool in stress reduction and elimination.

Just like regular exercise helps to reduce stress and keep your body healthy, regular meditation helps to reduce stress by exercising and keeping your mind healthy. Every day stress comes in many forms. It can begin with a hectic morning and impossible deadlines, it can continue with rush hour traffic, financial worries, parenting worries, relationship difficulties, coping with illness, etc. There really is no end to the list of possible sources of stress. While you may dislike the feeling of stress and challenge, it is important to keep in mind that challenges are a necessary part of life and personal growth. Without them, we never really have the opportunity to reach our full potential.

What meditation can help you achieve is the ability to see this challenges from a different perspective. You might learn to not sweat the small stuff, and to see the larger stuff as opportunities for gratitude rather than opportunities to destroy your emotional and physical health through stress. Meditation has become so recognized as a stress reducing tool, that the majority of therapists are open to teaching it as a way to help their patients reduce the impact of stress on their lives. Using meditation as a means to treat stress can improve interpersonal relationships, help you to become a better parent and/or coworker, and reduce the likelihood of burnout in both your personal and professional lives.

Before we can really understand how meditation can help ease stress, we must first really understand what stress is. Stress itself is highly subjective. It might mean something different to each of us.

So, how exactly can we define it? The best and simplest way of defining stress is to simply say that it is an emotional and physiological response to change. Notice here that I said change and not challenge. This is because of the way we interpret those two words. We can see change as being a positive, but see challenge as being overwhelmingly negative.

The fact is that all change, even positive and welcomed change, poses some challenges, and our bodies are going to react to those challenges whether we are enjoying them or not. Have you ever undergone a period of adjustment in your life caused by wonderful and wanted changes? Graduation, marriage, the welcoming of a child into your home, etc. are all examples of changes we often seek to bring about ourselves, but still can cause a great deal of stress. Stress is sometimes sneaky, letting you feel as though you are handling things well without a bit of stress, only to accumulate behind the scenes and leave you in a messy ball of stress at some unexpected point down the road.

Regardless of the type of stress you are experiencing, or how high your threshold appears to be for stress inducing events, stress has an incredible negative impact on your body. Stress responses are produced in the sympathetic nervous system, which is responsible for the fight or flight response and it is also responsible for the good types of "stress" such as the fluttering in your stomach before a first kiss. On the opposite side of the sympathetic nervous system is the parasympathetic nervous system, which is what balances the fight or flight response and returns the body to a normal balanced state.

When we become chronically stressed, the parasympathetic system becomes overwhelmed and does not have the opportunity to produce the proper recovery response.Research measured the physiological effects of stress on animals and you might be surprised at what they found. When introduced to various types of stressful stimuli from bright lights to loud noises and other sensory stressors, the animals always had the same physiological effects that included the enlargement of adrenal glands, stomach ulcerations and the shrinking of lymphatic tissue. Over time, repetitive stress caused serious health conditions such as inflammatory diseases, heart disease, stroke and kidney disease. It became obvious that stress has long term, dire consequences.

Aside from the health implications of chronic stress, when we are stressed we are also more likely to react poorly, behave inappropriately and make bad decisions. What does this do for us? For most of us a continued pattern of bad choices is only going to lead to even greater stress. The cycle can be vicious and never ending, that is unless you choose to do something about it.

When you use meditation to address the stress in your life what you are really doing is taking ownership and responsibility for your emotional state and your mental reactions to stressful stimuli. Through meditation practice, you learn to cultivate perspective and response. Rather than letting stress happen to you, you learn how to react and how to produce outcomes that are desirable and healthy. You become more aware, or mindful, of your experiences, you learn to recognize destructive patterns and you can train yourself to visualize the outcome you desire, the outcome that is most in line with your true happiness, and help to make it a reality.

Stress is reduced by meditation because your awareness and full vision of the situation gives you the opportunity to make choices. You are no longer a victim of the circumstance, but instead the one in charge, the one who can determine the outcome and choose to experience positivity and growth from every challenge rather than let it deteriorate your quality of life and long term health.

Meditation for stress is not difficult, and is not time consuming. Just a few minutes a day can help change how you are experiencing your life. One way that meditation can be especially useful for stressful events is by learning how to take mini meditation breaks. Once youhave begun a regular meditation practice and have become familiar with how to get your body relaxed, you can then take those techniques and use them in shorter five to ten minute sessions whenever you are feeling overwhelmed with stress. A few minutes before a meeting, while you are stopped in rush hour traffic, before or after that serious conversation with a loved one, before a big presentation. Meditation is more effective than medicine because you can take it anywhere, administer it whenever you want and in whatever dosage you feel is necessary. Meditation takes the control away from stress and places it back in your hands.

Meditation and Depression

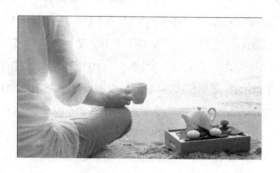

In the United States, nearly seven percent of the adult population over the age of eighteen experiences clinical depression. This is a statistic based only on what we know. That truth is that there are thousands of people who suffer depression silently, never seeking the diagnosis from a trained medical professional and never seeking treatment of any kind. This might be because of lack of available medical care, it might be because of the stigma associated with depression or it might be that when someone is depressed, sometimes caring enough about yourself to seek help can be overwhelming.

Depression can be situational or organic in nature. This means that in some cases depression is caused by external factors such as a major, unwelcomed change. Situations such as divorce, illness, death of a loved one, job loss, empty nest syndrome and financial worries are all examples of situational depression. Organic depression is an imbalance of chemicals in the brain which causes depressive thoughts and behaviors. There are basically two types of depression. One is temporary, the type of depression that is caused by an unpleasant event that you are eventually able to heal yourself from without the depressive thoughts consuming you for weeks on end. On the other side, we have clinical depression.

According to the Mayo Clinic, clinical depression is characterized by experiencing at least five of the following symptoms, most of the day, every day, for a period of two weeks or greater:

• Depressed mood, such as feeling sad, empty or tearful (in children and teens, depressed mood can appear as constant irritability)

• Significantly reduced interest or feeling no pleasure in all or most activities

• Significant weight loss when not dieting, weight gain, or decrease or increase in appetite (in children, failure to gain weight as expected)

• Insomnia or increased desire to sleep

• Either restlessness or slowed behavior that can be observed by others

• Fatigue or loss of energy

• Feelings of worthlessness, or excessive or inappropriate guilt

• Trouble making decisions, or trouble thinking or concentrating

• Recurrent thoughts of death or suicide, or a suicide attempt

Many times when someone reaches out to a medical professional with concerns of depression, they are treated with pharmaceuticals. Some of these medications can be very beneficial for certain people. However, like all medications, they come with their own list of unpleasant side effects. But more importantly is that not every medication works for every person. Many people end up trying several anti depressant medications in an effort to find the one that helps them regain the balance in their life only to discover that medication and have it quit working two years down the road. This is another issue with the automatic medication process. We end up treating the symptoms of depression, but seldom the cause.

Because depression is so individual, you cannot say that meditation will heal all depression. What we can say is that for the majority of people who are willing to try and devote a small portion of their day, that the severity of their depressive symptoms will lessen, they will experience fewer or less severe depressive episodes, and they can accomplish this with or without additional medications. Even with this, it is important that if you are experiencing depression that you talk to a professional about what you are going through. This book is not intended to replace professional therapy or remedies, nor is it an alternate self treatment guide.

Learning to meditate while depressed can be challenging, but well worth it. If you have experienced depression, then you know how difficult it can be to gain the energy to focus positively on anything. When you are depressed, your resources are tapped, you feel empty like you have nothing left to give, not even to yourself. When you are beginning to meditate, you might feel that it is a hopeless endeavor. For this reason, if you are beginning meditation while you are clinically depressed, be extra gentle on yourself in the beginning. For example, rather than trying to devote thirty minutes to absolute mindfulness each day, try starting with ten minutes of concentrated breathing, focusing only on the breath entering and leaving your body, rather than on mindful and focused thoughts.

Eventually, you can increase the "intensity" of your meditative practice by choosing to address your depressive thoughts and feelings. As you begin to do this, two things will happen. The first is that you will begin to realize that you have choices in how you react and feel. This can be overwhelming at first. The idea that you are responsible for your reactions and emotions is a huge and life changing concept. Secondly, you begin to train your mind how to look at things differently. Maybe meditation can't change brain chemistry to the point that it can heal depression completely, but in combination with other therapies, meditation can give you the ability to control how much depression affects your life and relationships.

Meditation and Anxiety

Everyone feels some degree of stress and anxiety from time to time. This is a normal aspect of life that serves a valuable function. But what do you do when feelings of fear and anxiety fill your life to a point that those negative emotions interfere with the daily aspects of your life, constantly leaving you feeling as though your world could fall apart at any moment. When anxiety reaches beyond intermittent episodes that occur after stressful events, it might be that you are actually suffering from General Anxiety Disorder or GAD. It is estimated that nearly 7 million American Adults suffer from some degree of GAD. This condition can be all encompassing with symptoms that include excessive worry, irrational fears, panic, self doubt, sleep disturbances, compulsive behaviors, flashbacks of unpleasant events and physiological symptoms such as rapid heartbeat, indigestion and muscle tension.

With GAD, reasonable worry is replaced with irrational fears, often about imagined events. Just like with stress and depression, there is also a physical side of anxiety. Anxiety will often keep you awake at night and cause long lasting sleep disturbances. Lack of proper sleep over extended periods of time can cause problems in your personal and professional life, but also can have serious health implications. Sleep disturbances have been linked to cardiac disease including heart attacks and stroke. Like any mental disorder, it is important to speak with a health professional about your symptoms, however along with that there are natural care remedies that you can use as tools against anxiety, one of which is meditation.

When you are anxious, your mind is usually racing. Thoughts run through at a mile of minute. Meditation is the perfect approach for quieting an overactive mind. If you suffer from anxiety then you know just how difficult it can be to train your mind to be quiet and focused in a place of serenity rather than fear. When beginning meditation while coping with GAD, the best approach is to start with short sessions. Often times, people with GAD find it easier to begin with guided meditations which help to serve as a type of distraction from obsessive thoughts that are sometimes associated with GAD.

Once you can take your mind from a place of anxiety and fear, and focus in short bouts of guided meditation, you will begin to feel relief from your symptoms. As your meditation practice grows, and your sessions begin to lengthen, you will notice that less and less of your day is consumed with fearful thoughts. As you begin to heal, through meditation you can train your mind to give less attention to the parts responsible for anxious thoughts over a period of six to eight weeks.

No matter if you suffer from anxiety, stress or depression or have other reasons for being interested in beginning meditative practice, you can make changes and experience life in ways that will have you on the path to balance, harmony and peace.

Chapter 18: Medications And Treatment

For Anxiety

It is very important that one must be available with the knowledge of options that he is available in order to treat anxiety disorders. This section aims to focus on how different medication and treatment approaches can be made use of in order to treat anxiety disorders. The kind of treatment your doctor will advise you will depend upon your diagnosis majorly. It is best that you begin with a talking treatment before moving on to medications. This is also recommended by the National Institute for Health and Care Excellence (NICE). Let us now look at the different options available that can be used as a treatment:

Talking Treatments:

Talking treatments are also referred to as counseling or therapy sessions. These are a process in which you get to work with a trained and professional therapist in order to understand the causes and solutions of your anxiety. There are several different kinds of talking treatments available all around.

However, the most commonly used treatment for managing anxiety is cognitive-behavioral therapy (CBT). So, what exactly is the cognitive behavioral therapy? CBT is a specific type of talking treatment that aims to signify and highlight the connections between one's cognitions, feelings as well as behavior. The aim is to help individuals develop practical skills in order to manage these in more positive ways.

Self-help resources

What are the self-help resources? Self-help resources are resources that have been come up with by health care professionals in order to help manage anxiety. These resources can come in different forms, including computer programs or workbooks. Computer programs can include some such as Fearfighter.

A fearfighter is a CBT computer-based program useful for the treatment of panic, anxiety as well as phobias. The program is freely available upon prescription through the NHS. There are many people who prefer the use of CCBT before they see a therapist in person. In order to have access to self-resources, individuals can buy self-help workbooks from different bookshops and specialist organizational websites. They can make use of their local library to order specific self-help books that can be borrowed for free.

Applied Relaxation Therapy

This form of treatment revolves around learning how to relax one's muscles in situations where normally anxiety is experienced. Applied relaxation therapy should be made use of and delivered by a trained therapist- usually for a session that is carried out every week for a period of about three to four months. You are more likely to be prescribed the use of applied relaxation therapy if you are diagnosed with generalized anxiety disorder or agoraphobia.

Exercising on Prescription

You can be prescribed exercise for several different problems, and these include mental health issues. If you are prescribed exercise, then you must try to refer to a qualified trainer who can help you set up an exercise program that can suit you and your requirements.

Medications might sometimes form part of your treatment. Your doctor might feel the need to prescribe you some medication in order to help you manage your anxiety well. The types of medication that can be used to manage anxiety are four, and these include antidepressants, beta-blockers, tranquilizers, and an anticonvulsant drug; the pregabalin. Let us look at each of these different type of medication in more detail:

Antidepressants

Antidepressants help individuals feel calmer and abler to take advantage of another treatment, such as the one known as talking treatment. Antidepressants that are most commonly prescribed for anxiety conditions include selective serotonin reuptake inhibitors such as citalopram (Celexa), fluoxetine (Prozac), escitalopram (Lexapro), paroxetine (Paxil) and sertraline (Zoloft). All these medications tend to relieve symptoms of anxiety by blocking the reabsorption of serotonin by the nerve cells within the brain. This results in more levels of serotonin being available, which improves and enhances neurotransmission; the sending of nerve impulses and improves the mood of the individual.

There are some antidepressants known as the tricyclic antidepressants such as imipramine, amitriptyline, and nortriptyline — these work to inhibit the reabsorption of the neurotransmitter's norepinephrine and serotonin. If no benefits are derived from a certain antidepressant after a time period of about three months, doctors suggest and recommend another antidepressant to their patients. Some people answer and respond well to one drug and do not respond well to the other. It is very common for people to try two or more antidepressant drugs before they can find the one that works best for them.

Tranquilizers

You might be prescribed to use tranquilizers (benzodiazepines) if the intensity of your anxiety is very strong or disabling. Tranquilizers do not work to tackle the cause of your anxiety but can bring some amount of relief until you are prescribed with some other treatment possible. Tranquilizers are supposed to be a temporary measure because addiction to these drugs is highly possible, which can result in difficulty to withdraw. Benzodiazepines promote and encourage relaxation and reduce muscular tension as well as other physical symptoms of anxiety. These are often used for short-term management of anxiety, such as for minor medical processes and procedures.

Beta-Blockers

Beta-blockers such as propranolol can cure and treat various physical symptoms of anxiety such as palpitations, rapid heartbeat, and shaking (tremor). However, these aren't psychiatric medications, and so they won't work to reduce any of your psychological symptoms.

Other medications for anxiety include MAOI's, which are the monoamine oxidase inhibitors, anticonvulsants, and atypical antipsychotics. In case of any side-effects that you experience from any medication, make sure to contact your physician. Do not stop taking medication abruptly as this can create more health risks and problems.

Chapter 19: Commit Your Two Minutes

Each Day

What can happen in two minutes? Allot two minutes each day. This strategy will help in reducing your stress and anxiety and boost your self-confidence.

Did you know that the most influential leaders in the world have higher levels of testosterone? This condition gives a person a higher level of confidence. These leaders also have lower levels of cortisol, which help in giving them a better grasp of stress and the ability to handle anxiety and pressure.

You don't have to be a leader in order to have these traits, but there is nothing wrong about thinking and acting like one. You simply have to learn the right ways that you can do to increase the levels of your testosterone and lower your system's cortisol levels.

Where did the concept come from? This is a result of the research from reputable institutions and universities, such as The University of Oregon, The University of Texas and Harvard University. The studies found out that when your body is able to maintain the right levels of hormones, your system becomes more confident, relaxed and assertive. You become more ready in handling stress and easily adapt to it.

How do you attain the right levels of testosterone and cortisol? The levels of these hormones change in a fast manner depending on the physical, social and environmental factors that you are exposed to. No matter what you are surrounded with, you can still maintain the proper balance of the levels of these hormones by having the right body posture.

Your body language influences the levels of your hormones and your confidence. This is what Amy Cuddy, a researcher from Harvard University, and her team, found out after conducting a series of experiments.

The research classified body positions into two categories – the high power poses that are open and relaxed and the low power poses that are guarded and closed. The research came up with this conclusion. The high power poses are able to increase testosterone levels by 20 percent, which translates to increased confidence, and decrease the cortisol levels by 25 percent that works by reducing a person's anxiety.

The Two-Minute Habit

Are you aware of "The Wonder Woman" pose? You can try searching for an image of the hero online and look closely at her pose. It is the most popular high power pose.

It is easy to do. Stand tall with your chin up and chest out. Put your hands on your hips. Maintain the pose for two minutes. Regardless of what the pose is called, this can still be done no matter what your gender is.

It is up to you when you would want to do the pose, but make sure that you do every day for at least two minutes. There are some people who escape from their busy schedules for several minutes. They perform this pose along with other breathing exercises in order to alleviate stress and feel recharged. You can also do this at the beginning of your day. You can combine this with other exercises and meditation.

Boosting your confidence doesn't end here, but it helps a lot. Try doing the two-minute high power pose before proceeding with your job interview or presentation. Do this before leaving the house to attend a social gathering. You will immediately feel the difference.

Your effort doesn't end here. You are a work in progress. This is an additional strategy that can help you in dealing with anxiety. Always think like a leader. Aside from having a focused mental state, you must also show your confidence through your body posture.

Watch Ted Talk about the Wonder Woman Pose for more information: https://www.youtube.com/watch?v=Ks-_Mh1QhMc

Chapter 20: Tips For Anxiety Relief

Worrying may be useful when it invites you to take actions and resolve a problem. However if you're preoccupied with bad-case scenarios, anxiousness may become a problem. Acute worrying is a psychological practice that needs to be taken care. You can guide your mind to be calm and see life from an optimistic view point.

What is the problem, stop worrying

Regularly worrying keeps you awake at night, make you anxious and nervous in during the day. The point is what is the problem, quit worrying.

In most persistent worriers, the worrying feelings are powered by attitude—both positive and negative.

The negative aspect, you might think that your regular worrying is destructive, that it's going to make you mad and may hamper your physical well-being. You may also worry that you will lose all your control over non-stop worrying.

On the positive side, you may believe that your worrying keeps you away from bad things, stops problems, prepares you for the worst, or can lead to solutions.

A negative belief increases your anxiety level and keeps you worried. However positive beliefs for worrying may also be as harmful. It's hard to quit the habit of worry if you think that the worrying guards you. So as to avoid worry and stress for good, you should give up the idea that the purpose of worrying is to provides a positive function. Once you feel that worrying or anxiousness is the dilemma, and not the answer, you can get back the control of your bothered mind.

Step I: Generate a worry period

It's hard to be dynamic in your everyday life when worry and stress are controlling your thoughts. You might have tried many things, from trying to think positive, analyzing your worries or distracting yourself, but nothing appears to work.

Why is it difficult to stop anxious thoughts

Forcing yourself to discontinue worrying doesn't work for long. You can divert yourself or repress your anxious thoughts for some time, but you can't drive them out for good. Indeed, when you try to do that, you only make them constant and stronger.

However, this doesn't mean that you cannot do anything to control your worry. You need to try a dissimilar approach. Now, here comes the need for the strategy of delaying worrying. Instead of trying to quit or get rid of a worried thought, you need to give yourself authorization to have it, but postpone your thinking about it.

How to delay worrying:

1.Generate a "worry period."

You need to choose a place and time for worrying. Please make sure that it remains the same each day (for example. in the bed room from 6:00 to 6:30 p.m.) and may be a bit early so that it will not make you worried just prior to you bedtime. During the period of worry, you can be worried for whatever comes in your mind. Apart from this will be a period free of all worries.

2.Delay your worry.

During the day, if a worry or a troubled thought comes in your mind then just write it on a piece of paper and delay it for the period dedicated for worries.Tell yourself that you will have a dedicated time to think about this later, so don't worry about this as of now. Do it later and perform your daily routine work.

3.Go through the "worry list" ONLY during the dedicated period for worries.

Have a look on all the worries that you noted down throughout the day. In case the worries are still disturbing you, you may think about them, but make sure it is limited only for the time you've allotted for the worry period. In case the worries don't seem to be important any further, make the worry period shorter and enjoy pleasure during the remaining part of the day.

As you cultivate an ability to delay or postpone your concerned thoughts, you'll begin to know that you have build more control over your anxiousness and worries than you think.

Step II: Inquire yourself if there is solution to the problem

Running over the problem in your head divert you from your emotions and makes you feel like you're getting something accomplished. But worrying and problem solving are two separate things.

Problem solving involves assessing a situation, coming up with tangible steps for dealing with it, and then putting it into action. On the other hand, worrying barely leads to solutions.

Difference between solvable and unsolvable worries

If a worry start bothering you, you may ask yourself a question that whether this problem is something you can really solve.

Useful, resolvable worries are the ones which can be action upon immediately. For example, in case you're bothered about your invoices, you may call the crediting company to check about any payment options that are flexible as per your budget. Useless, unsolvable worries can be termed as the ones for which we do not have any related action. "What if I meet with an accident?"

You can start brainstorming, if the worry is resolvable. Prepare a list of almost all the available and thinkable solutions that come in your mind.Concentrate on the problems which comes under your direct authority, in place of the realities and circumstances that are uncontrollable. After you've assessed your possibilities, prepare an action plan. Once the plan has been prepared start working a little on the worries, and your anxiousness would also reduce.

Step III: Accept insecurity

The helplessness to tolerate insecurity plays a big role in dealing with your worries and anxiety.Acute worriers can't stand impulsiveness. They want to understand with hundred percent certainties that what will happen in future. Worrying can be considered as a prediction on what is stored in future for us — an option to get rid of unfriendly surprises and have control on the results. The only problem is, it doesn't works.

Just thinking and getting worried for the items that may go wrong doesn't make your life predictable in any way. You may feel safe when you're worrying, but it's just a delusion. Concentrating on worst-case circumstances would not avoid the worst things from actually happening in your life. It would only restrict you from actually enjoying your present which has certain good things for you.So, if you are willing to get rid of your worries, you should initiate by attacking your requirement for immediate answers and certainty.

Step IV: Challenge fearful opinions

If you undergo an acute anxiety and anxiousness, there are possibilities that you may start looking this world in more dangerous way than it is in reality. As an example, you might jump directly in worst-case situations, or take every harmful thoughts as if they were in reality. You might also disgrace your abilities to take care life's problems, assuming you may fail on just receiving first impression of problem. These pessimistic, illogical, approaches are called cognitive distortions.

Cognitive distortions are not so easy to quit.Often, they become an integral part of your life and may become so reflex that you're not even aware of the situation. To quit these thinking habits, anxiety and worry you must rehabilitate your mind.

Start by recognizing the terrifying thought in a lot of details about what worries or frighten you. After that, instead of analyzing your feelings as truth, you may handle them as hypotheses you're testing out. The more you study and confront your doubts and worries; you'll build a more objective perspective.

Step V: Be alert how others influence you

Studies show that we easily "catch" moods of other people—also from an unfamiliar person who never speaks a word.

You may not realize how people or circumstances affect you. Perhaps this is how it's always happening in your family, or you've been facing the stressful situations for so long that it feels normal now. You can keep a worry diary for a week or so. Whenever you feel worry, note down the feelings and what activate it.

Spend a lesser amount of time with those who make you worried. Is there some person in your life who always make you feel stressed or pulls you down or? You should spend less time with that person.

Select your confidantes cautiously. You should know whom to talk to about your situations that make you worried. Several people can help you to increase your outlook, while some will feed into your fears, worries and stress.

Step VI: Follow mindfulness

Worrying mainly focus on your future—on what might can happen and what you'll do in regard to it. By bringing your awareness back to the present, you can be free from your worries.

Admit and observe your worried beliefs and feelings. Don't try to overlook, fight, or manage them like you generally would. Instead, simply examine them as if from an outsider's viewpoint, without any reaction.

Allow your worries to go. Observe that when you don't try to direct the concerned thoughts that come up, they soon pass away, like smoke moving in the air. It's only when you hold your worries that you get caught.

Stay focused on present. Be attentive to the feelings of your body, the pace while you breathe, the feelings that flow in your mind and your changing emotions. When you get stuck on some specific thought, divert your thoughts to the today.

Use of mindfulness introspection to stay concentrated on today is a very simple theory, however it asks for a lot of practice and hard work to fetch the advantages.Initially, you may identify that your thoughts keep on taking a U-turn towards your worries. You need to avoid frustration.Every time you bring your concentration back to today, you are emphasizing a new psychological routine that would help you get rid a negative worry cycle full of negativity.

Chapter 21: Set Yourself Up With

Rewards

So you have done your part reviewing and you feel that you are ready to take the exam. Now is as good a time as any to take a breather and relax.

Relaxing is a form of reward that you give yourself to allow yourself to regroup and ease jangled nerves. This is because for most people, gearing up for an exam is a battle worse than taking the exam itself. They become hard on themselves, stretching the limit of what they are capable of. In the process they get worn out, at times even burned out. This does not bode well on either a physical or mental level. When brought to the extreme, stress can weaken the body's immune system, making it easier to get victimized by illnesses of all sort. On a mental level, stress can cause unnecessary anxiety, which could affect the way you take or handle the exam. Either way, it is a losing proposition for you.

Granted that going over notes and reviewing lessons is difficult, there are things that you can do to motivate yourself to work harder and be better. Yes, this involves rewarding yourself for having done much work. This will help you keep things in perspective while staying committed to the goals you have laid out at the beginning.

These goals should indicate what you intend to accomplish over a given period of time. Moreover, these goals should serve as a guide as you prepare for the actual exam. Once done reviewing, assess your goals and see if they have been met. If yes, then a little reward will affirm your commitment to your goals and in the process make you feel more confident.

These rewards need not be extravagant. In fact, they can be simple pleasures that you can use to make yourself a little better. A bar of dark chocolate? Why not. A steaming bowl of dimsum from your favorite Chinese diner? Sure. A movie perhaps? You deserve it.

The confidence you get out of this simple exercise will help you conquer your apprehensions during the exam. The knowledge that comes from the fact that you have spent considerable time and exerted energy to prepare should serve as a little incentive as you begin answering the questions.

Once you are done with the exam, do not make the common mistake of dwelling excessively on it. Instead, move on and brace yourself with the resources and tools you need for the next exam. Trying to nitpick the exam by discussing what the answers are is bound to yield feelings of self-doubt if your answers are different, or a false sense of security if you have common answers. The fact is, you will not know how you fared until the scores are out, but you can still feel good about yourself if you are confident that you have indeed done well.

In the end, exams should be treated not as mere academic requirements to pass, but as challenges to surpass and learn from. In fact, when set in the context of how they help define who you are and what your character is, they can be great tools for learning, too. Therefore, exams should not be a source of fear, anxiety, or frustration. Nor should they be treated with mechanical predisposition. Treat them as a great starting point for learning. As such, developing the right attitude and mindset is crucial in making each exam count.

Chapter 22: Massage

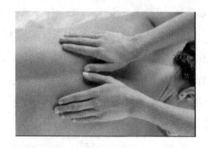

Massage triggers various actions in the body: accelerates the elimination of toxins, stimulates blood circulation, relieves sore muscles and creates a feeling of pleasure. Tact is a fundamental form of communication and a massage shared between partners can transmit confidence, especially in times of stress. A basic massage does not require expertise because it does not interfere with any internal organ of the body. A traditional massage uses three main features: rubbing or caressing, light pressure and beats. The first two are the most common when performing a traditional massage.

Before giving a massage, the two partners need to spend a couple of minutes relaxing before starting the massage, because the tension of the person that is going to give the massage can be easily transmitted to the person that is receiving it.

Here is how you can prepare yourself and your partner to enjoy 100% of the massage experience:

-Start the massage by warming your hands and resting them in the person for some time to make contact. Then rub the hands with a pleasing oil aroma so you can perform firm and uniform movements.

-Keep contact with the skin so that the massage is felt as a continuous floating movement.

-Put more oil on a warm plate placed near so you can dip a hand in it without having to change the pace.

-Change the pressure in different areas of the body to increase interest.

-Slow down as you reach the end of the massage, leaving your hands to rest in the same position for about a minute.

-The areas around the upper body are more prone to stress: shoulders, arms, neck and forehead.

-Massage for about 20 minutes and then rest for a while to maximize sensation.

-Give special attention to any areas where you feel stiff muscles. Press them with the thumbs and palms, and rub the areas around them to encourage the removal of impurities. Avoid pressing force directly on the spine.

In Western society today, massage is widely accepted and regularly used by many people as a complement to conventional medicine. You can even massage your own forehead and neck, a quick way to revitalize or stress relief from a headache. But if a specialized friend or partner give you a massage, it can become a treatment for the whole body.

Massaging the Forehead

-Place both hands in the center of the forehead of the person, with fingertips touching each other.

-Move your hands in two directions: upward, toward the root of the hair, and down, towards the cheekbones. Use long firm strokes, one after the other in a nearly circular line. Repeat several times.

-Finish the sequence with your hands resting on the forehead of the receiver for a few seconds.

-Apply more oil and put your hands on the forehead of the person again, this time one over the other.

-With large movements, move your hands up, towards the hairline.

-Keep the continuous movement, with one hand to replace the other.

-Repeat several times and then finish putting the hands at rest. Ask for feedback.

Massage of the Neck and Shoulders

-Place your hands on the neck just below the ears, and in continuous motion, move your hands over the shoulders, stopping when you reach the upper arms.

-Repeat several times and finish with your hands resting on the starting position. The person should feel that the tension in the neck and shoulders have disappeared.

-Apply more oil and start with hands placed at the end of the neck, near the shoulders, palms cupped over the muscle.

-Keep your hands in contact with your shoulders, use the flat part of the thumb to press the area on the back of the neck, in circular motion. Do not apply direct pressure on the spine.

-Takes all the time that necessary as long as the person feel comfortable.

Massage of the Arms

-With the person's arm face down on a towel, put your hands in the back of the arm and slide down from the shoulder to the elbow using a steady motion.

-Separate your hands and let them slip down, pressing the back of the forearm.

-Using both hands, press the back of the forearm from the wrist to the elbow. Repeat the sequence in the upper arm.

-Massage the elbow with a circular motion. Use a lot of oil, as this area can be dry.

-Ask the person to raise the forearm and use your thumbs to press the front of the forearm, from the wrist to the elbow. Repeat several times.

-Complete by giving lightly massage from the shoulder to the fingertips. Repeat on the other arm.